About Rails-to-Trails Conservancy

Headquartered in Washington, D.C., Rails-to-Trails Conservancy (RTC) is a nonprofit organization dedicated to building a nation connected by trails. RTC reimagines public spaces to create safe ways for everyone to walk, bike, and be active outdoors.

Railways helped build America. Spanning from coast to coast, these ribbons of steel linked people, communities, and enterprises, spurring commerce and forging a single nation that bridges a continent. But in recent decades, many of these routes have fallen into disuse, severing communal ties that helped bind Americans together.

When RTC opened its doors in 1986, the rail-trail movement was in its infancy. Most projects, created for recreation and conservation, focused on single, linear routes in rural areas. RTC sought broader protection for the unused corridors, incorporating rural, suburban, and urban routes.

Year after year, RTC's efforts to protect and align public funding with trail building created an environment that allowed trail advocates in communities across the country to initiate projects. The ever-growing ranks of these professionals, volunteers, and RTC supporters have built momentum for the national rail-trails movement. As the number of supporters has multiplied, so have the rail-trails.

Americans now enjoy more than 25,000 miles of open rail-trails, and as they flock to the trails to connect with family members and friends, enjoy nature, and access places in their local neighborhoods and beyond, their economic prosperity, health, and overall well-being continue to flourish.

A signature endeavor of RTC is **TrailLink.com™,** America's portal to these rail-trails and other multiuse trails. When we launched the website in 2000, RTC was one of the first organizations to compile such detailed trail information on a national scale. Today, TrailLink.com continues to play a critical role in both encouraging and satisfying the country's growing need for opportunities to use trails for recreation or transportation. This free trail-finder database—which includes detailed descriptions, interactive maps, photo galleries, and firsth   —can be used as a companion resource to this gui

With a grassroots community more th
committed to ensuring a better future for Ar
and the connections they inspire. Learn mo

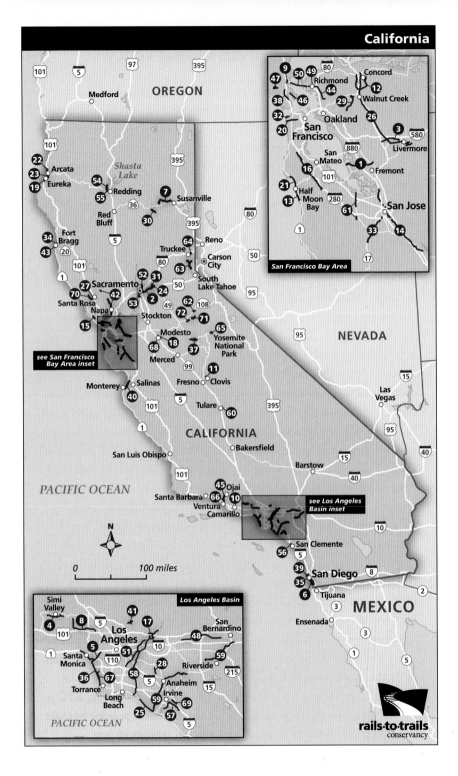

California

101 5 97 395

Medford OREGON

San Francisco Bay Area

9 49 80
47 50 Richmond Concord
  44 12
38 46 29 Walnut Creek
32 Oakland 26
20 San 3 580
  Francisco Livermore
  San 880
  Mateo 1
16 Fremont
21 101
13 Half 280
  Moon San Jose
  Bay 61
1 33 14
  17

101
22 Arcata Shasta
23 Lake
19 Eureka 395
54
55 Redding 7
  36 Susanville
Red 30
Bluff 395
34 Fort 80
43 Bragg 5 Reno
20 Truckee 64
1 101 Carson
  52 31 City
  70 27 Sacramento 63 50
  42 24 South
  53 2 Lake Tahoe 95
Santa Rosa 49 62
15 Napa 72 108 NEVADA
  Stockton 71
  65
  Modesto 95
  68 18 Yosemite
Monterey Salinas Merced 37 National
40 99 Park 95
  11 Las
101 Fresno Clovis Vegas
  5
  Tulare 15
  60 395
  CALIFORNIA
  Bakersfield
San Luis Obispo Barstow 15 40
  101 40
PACIFIC OCEAN 45 Ojai 10
Santa Barbara 66 10
  Ventura
  Camarillo see Los Angeles
  Basin inset
see San Francisco
Bay Area inset

N

0 100 miles

  San Clemente
  56 5
  39 San Diego 8
  35
  6 Tijuana 2
  MEXICO
  3
  Ensenada
  3
  1 5

Los Angeles Basin
Simi
Valley 41
4 8 5 17 San
101 Los Bernardino
  5 Angeles 48
1 Santa 51 10
  Monica 110 28 59
  58 Riverside
36 67 5 215
Torrance Anaheim 15
  Long Irvine 69
  Beach 59
  25 57 5
PACIFIC OCEAN

rails·to·trails
conservancy

iv

Table of Contents

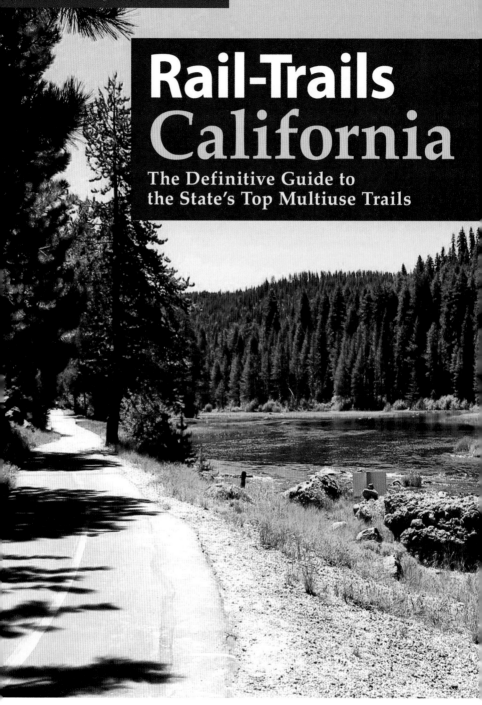

The Official Rails-to-Trails
Conservancy Guidebook

Rail-Trails
California

The Definitive Guide to
the State's Top Multiuse Trails

WILDERNESS PRESS ... *on the trail since 1967*

Rail-Trails: California
1st Edition
Copyright © 2023 by Rails-to-Trails Conservancy
Cover and interior photographs copyright © 2023 by Rails-to-Trails Conservancy

Project editor: Kate Johnson
Maps: Lohnes+Wright; map data © OpenStreetMap contributors
Cover design: Scott McGrew
Book design and layout: Annie Long
Proofreader: Emily Beaumont
Indexer: Rich Carlson

Library of Congress Cataloging-in-Publication Data
Names: Rails-to-Trails Conservancy author.
Title: Rail-trails : California : the definitive guide to the state's top multiuse trails /
  Rails-to-Trails Conservancy.
Description: 1st edition. | Birmingham, AL : Wilderness Press, 2023. |
  Includes index.
Identifiers: LCCN 2022055342 (print) | LCCN 2022055343 (ebook) |
  ISBN 9781643590875 (pbk.) | ISBN 9781643590882 (ebook)
Subjects: LCSH: Rail-trails—California—Guidebooks. | Trails—California—
  Guidebooks. | Hiking—California—Guidebooks. | Walking—California—
  Guidebooks. | Running—California—Guidebooks. | Cycling—California—
  Guidebooks. | California—Guidebooks.
Classification: LCC GV199.42.C2 R35 2023 (pbk.) | LCC GV199.42.C2 (ebook) |
  DDC 796.5109794—dc23/eng/20221117
LC record available at lccn.loc.gov/2022055342
LC ebook record available at lccn.loc.gov/2022055343

Published by: 🐾 **WILDERNESS PRESS**
An imprint of AdventureKEEN
2204 First Ave. S, Ste. 102
Birmingham, AL 35233
800-678-7006; fax 877-374-9016

Visit wildernesspress.com for a complete listing of our books and for ordering information. Contact us at our website, at facebook.com/wildernesspress1967, or at twitter.com
/wilderness1967 with questions or comments. To find out more about who we are and what
we're doing, visit blog.wildernesspress.com.

Printed in the United States of America
Distributed by Publishers Group West

Front cover photo: Tahoe City Public Utility District Multi-Use Trail System (see page 229);
photographed by TrailLink user sherstone; *Back cover photo:* Monterey Bay Coastal Recreation Trail (see page 147); photographed by Elizabeth Bean Photography

SAFETY NOTICE Although Wilderness Press and Rails-to-Trails Conservancy have made
every attempt to ensure that the information in this book is accurate at press time, they are
not responsible for any loss, damage, injury, or inconvenience that may occur to anyone while
using this book. You are responsible for your own safety and health while in the wilderness.
The fact that a trail is described in this book does not mean that it will be safe for you. Be aware
that trail conditions can change from day to day. Always check local conditions, know your
own limitations, and consult a map.

Welcome to the *Rail-Trails: California* guidebook, a comprehensive companion for discovering the state's top rail-trails and multiuse pathways. This book will help you uncover fantastic opportunities to get outdoors on California's trails—whether for exercise, transportation, or just pure fun.

Rails-to-Trails Conservancy's (RTC's) mission is to build a nation connected by trails. We reimagine public spaces to create safe ways for everyone to walk, bike, and be active outdoors. We hope this book will inspire you to experience firsthand how trails can connect people to one another and to the places they love, while also creating connections to nature, history, and culture.

Since its founding in 1986, RTC has witnessed massive growth in the rail-trail and active transportation movement. Today, more than 25,000 miles of completed rail-trails provide invaluable benefits for people and communities across the country. We hope you find this book to be a delightful and informative resource for discovering the many unique trail destinations throughout California.

I'll be out on the trails, too, experiencing the thrill of the ride right alongside you. Be sure to say hello and share your #TrailMoments with us on social media. You can find us @railstotrails on Facebook, Instagram, and Twitter. Participate in our Trail Moments initiative by sharing your stories of resilience, joy, health, and connection at **trailmoments.org**!

Enjoy the journey,

Ryan Chao, President, Rails-to-Trails Conservancy

Acknowledgments

Special acknowledgment is owed to Laura Stark and Amy Kapp, editors of this guidebook, and to Derek Strout and Bart Wright (with Lohnes+Wright) for their work on the creation of the trail maps included in the book. Rails-to-Trails Conservancy also thanks Gene Bisbee and Amy Ahn for their writing and editing assistance.

We also appreciate the following staff and intern contributors, as well as local trail managers, who helped us ensure that the maps, photographs, and trail descriptions are as accurate as possible.

Kevin Belle	Miguel Jiménez
Ken Bryan	Willie Karidis
Danielle Casavant	Ben Kaufman
Laura Cohen	Mary Ellen Koontz
Ryan Cree	Joe LaCroix
Peter Dean	Anthony Le
Cindy Dickerson	Suzanne Matyas
Andrew Dupuy	Kevin Mills
Noor Hannosh	Yvonne Mwangi
Brandi Horton	Eric Oberg
Brian Housh	Kelly Pack
Heather Irish	Anya Saretzky

Trail Number/Name	Page	Mileage	Walking	Cycling	Wheelchair Accessible	In-line Skating	Mountain Biking	Fishing	Horseback Riding	Cross-Country Skiing	Snowmobiling
1 Alameda Creek Regional Trails	9	24.4	●	●	●	●	●	●	●		
2 American River Parkway (Jedediah Smith Memorial Trail)	13	32	●	●	●	●		●			
3 Arroyo Mocho Trail	15	12.9	●	●	●	●	●				
4 Arroyo Simi Bike Path	19	8.6	●	●	●	●		●	●		
5 Ballona Creek Bike Path	21	6.4	●	●	●	●					
6 Bayshore Bikeway	25	17.1	●	●	●	●					
7 Bizz Johnson National Recreation Trail	29	25.4	●	●	●				●	●	●
8 Browns Creek Bike Path and Orange Line Bike Path	33	17.3	●	●	●	●					
9 Cal Park Hill Tunnel and SMART Pathway	35	2.5	●	●	●	●					
10 Calleguas Creek Bike Path	39	4.4	●	●	●	●					
11 Clovis Old Town Trail and Sugar Pine Trail	41	9.6	●	●	●	●					
12 Contra Costa Canal Regional Trail	45	13.8	●	●	●	●		●	●		
13 Cowell-Purisima Trail	49	4.1	●	●	●	●					
14 Coyote Creek Trail	53	25.6	●	●	●	●		●	●		
15 Cross Marin Trail	57	5.3	●	●	●				●		
16 Crystal Springs Regional Trail	61	16.5	●	●	●	●			●		
17 Donald and Bernice Watson Recreation Trail	65	1.6	●	●	●				●		
18 Dry Creek Trail (Peggy Mensinger Trail)	67	4.7	●	●	●	●					
19 Eureka Waterfront Trail	71	6.5	●	●	●	●		●			
20 Golden Gate Park Multiuse Trail	75	3.9	●	●	●	●					
21 Half Moon Bay Coastside Trail	79	7.5	●	●	●	●					
22 Hammond Trail	83	5.5	●	●	●			●	●		
23 Humboldt Bay Trail North	87	4.5	●	●	●	●					
24 Humbug–Willow Creek Trail	91	15	●	●	●	●					
25 Huntington Beach Bicycle Trail	95	8.3	●	●	●	●		●			

Trail Number/Name	Page	Mileage	Walking	Cycling	Wheelchair Accessible	In-line Skating	Mountain Biking	Fishing	Horseback Riding	Cross-Country Skiing	Snowmobiling
26 Iron Horse Regional Trail	99	32	●	●	●	●			●		
27 Joe Rodota Trail	103	8.5	●	●	●	●			●		
28 Juanita Cooke Greenbelt and Trail	107	2.5	●	●				●	●		
29 Lafayette-Moraga Regional Trail	109	7.7	●	●	●	●			●		
30 Lake Almanor Recreation Trail	113	11	●	●			●	●		●	
31 Lake Natoma Trail	117	5.5	●	●	●	●					
32 Lands End Trail	119	1.6	●				●				
33 Los Gatos Creek Trail	123	10.7	●	●	●	●					
34 MacKerricher Haul Road Trail	127	3.8	●	●	●			●	●		
35 Martin Luther King, Jr. Promenade	131	0.75	●		●						
36 Marvin Braude Bike Trail	133	22	●	●	●	●					
37 Merced River Trail	137	4.9	●				●	●			
38 Mill Valley/Sausalito Multiuse Pathway	141	3.7	●	●	●	●			●		
39 Mission Bay Bike Path	143	11.4	●	●	●	●					
40 Monterey Bay Coastal Recreation Trail	147	18	●	●	●	●			●		
41 Mt. Lowe Railway Trail	151	5.8	●				●		●		
42 Napa Valley Vine Trail	155	18.5	●	●	●	●					
43 Noyo Headlands Coastal Trail	159	4.5	●	●	●	●					
44 Ohlone Greenway	161	5.3	●	●	●	●					
45 Ojai Valley Trail	165	9.3	●	●	●	●			●		
46 Old Rail Trail	169	2.6	●	●	●	●					
47 Old Railroad Grade	173	4.4	●				●		●		
48 Pacific Electric Inland Empire Trail	175	20	●	●	●	●			●		
49 Richmond Greenway	179	2.5	●	●	●	●					

continued on next page

Trail Number/Name	Page	Mileage	Walking	Cycling	Wheelchair Accessible	In-line Skating	Mountain Biking	Fishing	Horseback Riding	Cross-Country Skiing	Snowmobiling
50 Richmond–San Rafael Bridge Path	183	6	•	•	•						
51 Rio Hondo River Trail	187	17.8	•	•	•	•			•		
52 Sacramento Northern Bikeway	191	10.1	•	•	•	•			•		
53 Sacramento River Parkway Trail	193	9.3	•	•	•	•					
54 Sacramento River Rail Trail	197	11.1	•	•	•	•		•			
55 Sacramento River Trail	201	12.3	•	•	•	•		•			
56 San Clemente Beach Trail	205	2.3	•	•	•			•			
57 San Diego Creek Trail	207	10.8	•	•	•	•					
58 San Gabriel River Trail	211	38	•	•	•	•					
59 Santa Ana River Trail	215	57.7	•	•	•	•			•		
60 Santa Fe Trail	219	5	•	•	•	•			•		
61 Stevens Creek Trail	221	5.9	•	•	•	•					
62 Sugar Pine Railway Trail	225	2.5	•				•			•	•
63 Tahoe City Public Utility District Multi-Use Trail System	229	18.7	•	•	•	•		•			
64 Truckee River Legacy Trail	233	4.8	•	•	•	•		•			
65 Valley Loop Trail	235	7.5	•	•	•	•		•			
66 Ventura River Trail	239	5.5	•	•	•	•					
67 Veterans Parkway	243	3.5	•		•						
68 Virginia Corridor Trailway	245	2.7	•	•	•	•					
69 Walnut Trail	249	3.4	•	•	•	•					
70 West County Regional Trail	251	5.5	•	•	•	•	•		•		
71 Westside Rails to Trails (Hull Creek to Clavey River)*	255	9	•	•					•		
72 Westside Rails to Trails (Tuolumne City to North Fork Tuolumne River)	257	5.5	•					•	•		

ATVs permitted on part of the trail

Of the more than 2,300 rail-trails across the country, 139 thread through California. These routes relate a two-part story: The first speaks to the early years of railroading, while the second showcases efforts by Rails-to-Trails Conservancy (RTC), other groups, and their supporters to resurrect these unused railroad corridors as public-use trails. This guidebook highlights 72 of the state's premier trails, including dozens of rail-trails and other multiuse pathways.

From a temperate rainforest to an arid desert, California offers a seemingly endless diversity of environments and landscapes to explore. Whether you feel at home along the beach or among the mountains, our country's most populous state probably has a trail experience tailored for you.

No list of the state's trails would be complete without the Bizz Johnson National Recreation Trail (page 29), an inductee into the Rail-Trail Hall of Fame (**railstotrails.org/halloffame**). The 25-mile pathway follows the Susan River Canyon through pine forestland between Westwood and a historical train depot at Susanville, traversing 12 bridges and two tunnels. Another not-to-miss experience in Northern California is a trip across the iconic Sundial Bridge along the Sacramento River Trail (page 201) in Redding.

No state has more national parks than California. Two trails in this book provide a scenic adventure through one of its most famous, Yosemite National Park, and its surrounding areas: the Valley Loop Trail—an easy, paved path departing right from the visitor center—and the ruggedly beautiful Merced River Trail.

For ocean lovers, a trail can't get much more picturesque than the Monterey Bay Coastal Recreation Trail, which hugs the water so closely that waves occasionally wash over it. Just north of that coastal pathway, the San Francisco Bay Area has no shortage of outdoor destinations and is home to a developing 2,600-miles-plus regional trail network being spearheaded by RTC and the Bay Area Trails Collaborative (**railstotrails.org/bay-area**) as a TrailNation™ project to increase safe walking, biking, and trail access for millions of Bay Area residents. One of the exciting projects in this vast trail system is the Napa Valley Vine Trail, a growing 47-mile route through California's North Coast wine region.

On the southern end of the state, the Bayshore Bikeway offers an eclectic mix of urban views of downtown San Diego and natural vistas of salt marshes and tidal flats as it winds nearly 270 degrees around San Diego Bay. And in Los Angeles, the iconic beachfront Marvin Braude Bike Trail—better known as The Strand by locals—may look familiar, as it's been featured in hundreds of TV shows and movies.

These are just a few of the gems you'll find in the Golden State, but no matter which route in *Rail-Trails: California* you decide to try, you're sure to find an experience to treasure.

What Is a Rail-Trail?

Rail-trails are multiuse public paths built along former railroad corridors. Most often flat or following a gentle grade, they are suited to walking, running, cycling, mountain biking, wheelchair use, in-line skating, cross-country skiing, and horseback riding. Since the 1960s, Americans have created more than 25,000 miles of rail-trails throughout the country.

These extremely popular recreation and transportation corridors traverse urban, suburban, and rural landscapes. Many preserve historical landmarks, while others serve as wildlife conservation corridors, linking isolated parks and establishing greenways in developed areas. Rail-trails also stimulate local economies by boosting tourism and promoting trailside businesses.

What Is a Rail-with-Trail?

A rail-with-trail is a public path that parallels a still-active rail line. Some run adjacent to fast-moving, scheduled trains, often linking public transportation stations, while others follow tourist routes and slow-moving excursion trains. Many share an easement, separated from the rails by fencing or other barriers. More than 400 rail-with-trails exist in 47 states across the country.

What Is the Rail-Trail Hall of Fame?

In 2007, RTC began recognizing exemplary rail-trails around the country through its Rail-Trail Hall of Fame. Inductees are selected based on merits such as scenic value, high use, trail and trailside amenities, historical significance, excellent management and maintenance of facilities, community connections, and geographic distribution. California boasts one Hall of Fame rail-trail: the Bizz Johnson National Recreation Trail (see page 29). For the full list of Hall-of-Fame rail-trails, visit **railstotrails .org/halloffame**.

What Is TrailNation™?

At RTC, we believe that communities are healthier and happier when trails are central to their design. Everything we love about trails gets better when we connect them, creating seamless trail networks that link neighborhoods, towns, cities, and entire regions together. That's why we're committed to connecting trails and building comprehensive trail systems that bring people together and get them where they want to go.

We've invested in eight TrailNation™ projects across the country—found in places that are diverse in their geography, culture, size, and scope—to prove what is possible when trail networks are central to our lives. One of these projects can be found in California: the developing Bay Area regional trail network, which is being spearheaded by the Bay Area Trails Collaborative and RTC to increase safe walking, biking, and trail access for millions of Bay Area residents. Look for the TrailNation logo throughout this book to find trails that are part of this exciting trail system. Learn more at **trailnation.org.**

About the Bay Area Trails Collaborative

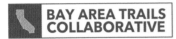

The vision of the Bay Area Trails Collaborative is to develop a 2,600-miles-plus regional trail network that will connect the San Francisco Bay Area in innovative new ways. Through the development of the trail network, the collaborative—currently made up of more than 50 organizations, agencies, and businesses—seeks to improve the overall quality of life in the region by creating more opportunities for recreation and active transportation, addressing health disparities in underserved communities, improving health and wellness, reducing pollution and greenhouse gases, and promoting environmental sustainability. Learn more at **railstotrails .org/bay-area.**

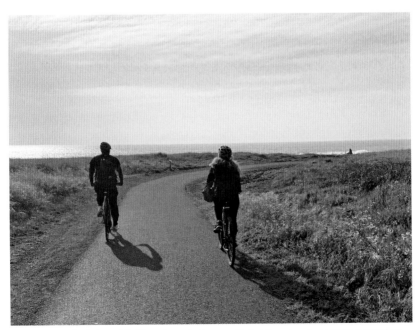

The Noyo Headlands Coastal Trail transformed a former mill site into a place for enjoying ocean views (see page 159). Brian Housh

Rail-Trails: *California* provides all the information you'll need to plan a rewarding trek on a rail-trail or other multiuse trail in the state. With words to inspire you and maps to chart your path, it makes choosing the best route a breeze. Following are some of the highlights.

Maps

You'll find two levels of maps in this book: a **state locator map** (see page iv) and **detailed trail maps**. Use these maps to find the trails nearest you, or select several neighboring trails and plan a weekend excursion. Once you find a trail on the state locator map, simply flip to the corresponding trail number for a full description. Accompanying trail maps indicate each route's access roads, trailheads, parking areas, restrooms, and other defining features.

Key to Map Icons

Parking

Drinking Water

Restrooms

Featured Trail

Connecting Trail

Active Railroad

Trail Descriptions

Trails are listed in alphabetical order. Each description begins with a summary of key facts about the trail, including possible uses. trail endpoints and mileage, a roughness rating, and the trail surface.

The map and summary information list the trail endpoints (either a city, street, or more specific location), with suggested start and finish points. Additional access points are marked on the maps and mentioned in the trail descriptions. The maps and descriptions also highlight available amenities, including parking; restrooms; and area attractions such as shops, services, museums, parks, and stadiums. Trail length is listed in miles, one way, and includes only completed trail; the mileage for any gaps in the trail will be noted in its description.

Each trail description includes a **roughness rating** from 1 to 3. A rating of 1 indicates a smooth, level surface that is accessible to users of all ages and abilities. A 2 rating means the surface may be loose and/or uneven and could pose a problem for road bikes and wheelchairs. A 3 rating suggests a rough surface that is recommended only for mountain bikers and hikers. Surfaces can range from asphalt or concrete to ballast, boardwalk, cinder, crushed stone, gravel, grass, dirt, sand, and/or wood chips. Where relevant, trail descriptions address alternating surface conditions.

All trails are open to pedestrians. Bicycles are permitted unless otherwise noted in the trail summary or description. The summary also indicates whether the trail is wheelchair accessible. Other possible uses include in-line skating, mountain biking, horseback riding, fishing, and cross-country skiing. While most trails are off-limits to motor vehicles, some local trail organizations do allow ATVs and snowmobiles.

Trail descriptions themselves suggest an ideal itinerary for each route, including the best parking areas and access points, where to begin, direction of travel, and any highlights along the way.

Each trail description also lists a local website for further information. Be sure to check these websites for updates and current conditions before you set out. **TrailLink.com** is another great resource for updated content on the trails in this guidebook.

Parking Waypoints

In the Parking section for each trail, we've included GPS coordinates for the main parking waypoints. These latitude and longitude coordinates can be used on a GPS device or in online mapping programs to locate parking areas. If you have a smartphone, you can use this guidebook along with Rails-to-Trails Conservancy's TrailLink app—available from the Apple App Store and Google Play—which provides driving directions at the tap of a waypoint.

Trail Use Guidelines

Rail-trails are popular destinations for a range of users, which makes them busy places to enjoy the outdoors. Following basic trail etiquette and safety guidelines will make your experience more pleasant.

➤ **Keep to the right,** except when passing.

➤ **Pass on the left, and give a clear, audible warning:** "On your left!"

➤ **Be aware of other trail users,** particularly around corners and blind spots, and be especially careful when entering a trail, changing direction, or passing so that you don't collide with traffic.

➤ **Respect wildlife and public and private property;** leave no trace and pack out litter.

➤ **Control your speed,** especially near pedestrians, playgrounds, and congested areas.

➤ **Travel single file.** Cyclists and pedestrians should ride or walk single file in congested areas or areas with reduced visibility.

➤ **Cross carefully at intersections;** always look both ways, and yield to through traffic. Pedestrians have the right-of-way.

➤ **Keep one ear open and your headphone volume low** to increase your awareness of your surroundings.

➤ **Wear a helmet and other safety gear** if you're cycling or in-line skating.

➤ **Consider visibility.** Wear reflective clothing, use bicycle lights, and bring flashlights or helmet-mounted lights for tunnel passages or twilight excursions.

➤ **Keep moving, and don't block the trail.** When taking a rest, move off the trail to the right. Groups should avoid congregating on or blocking the trails. If you have an accident on the trail, move to the right as soon as possible.

➤ **Bicyclists yield to all other trail users.** Pedestrians yield to horses. If in doubt, yield to all other trail users.

➤ **Dogs are permitted on most trails,** but some trails through parks, wildlife refuges, or other sensitive areas may not allow pets; it's best to check the trail website before your visit. If pets are permitted, keep your dog on a short leash and under your control at all times. Remove dog waste and place in a designated trash receptacle.

➤ **Teach your children these trail essentials,** and be diligent in keeping them out of faster-moving trail traffic.

➤ **Be prepared, especially on long-distance and rural trails.** Bring water, snacks, maps, a light source, matches, and other equipment you might need. Because some areas may not have good reception for mobile phones, know where you're going, and tell someone else your plan.

E-Bikes

Electric bicycles, commonly called e-bikes, are similar to standard bikes in appearance and operation but feature a small electric motor to assist the rider by adding power to the wheels. A three-tiered system has been developed to classify e-bikes based on speed capacity and other factors. Many states allow Class 1 (up to 20 mph; requires pedaling) and Class 2 (uses a throttle) e-bikes to operate on trails, but not Class 3 (up to 28 mph). However, these rules vary by local jurisdiction, so if you would like to ride an e-bike on one of the trails listed in this book, please visit the website listed for the trail or contact the local trail manager to determine whether the use of e-bikes is permitted. Learn more at **rtc.li/rtc-ebikes.**

Travel Precautions

When planning a trail excursion in the West, check wildfire risk levels before you go. Visit the website listed for the trail or contact the local trail manager to see if there are any fire restrictions in the area you plan to visit. You can also check regional or national resources, such as the Bureau of Land

Management (**blm.gov/programs/fire/fire-restrictions**), California Department of Forestry and Fire Protection (**fire.ca.gov**), or the **National Weather Service** (**weather.gov/fire**), for current wildfire assessments.

Another consideration in California and elsewhere are encampments of unhoused individuals along some trails, particularly in urban centers. If you come across an encampment, please keep a respectful distance and keep an eye out for individuals, pets, and wildlife that may be crossing the pathway from either side.

Due to California's significantly higher-than-average rainfall in late 2022 and early 2023, we also recommend that you plan ahead and check for any trail repair/closure notices on the trail's website or with the trail manager. You can also visit the National Weather Service website (**weather.gov/safety/flood -states-ca**) for local flood-hazard information; search by specific cities near the bottom of the web page. Additionally, if the trail you'd like to use runs through land managed by the California Department of Parks and Recreation, such as a state park or state beach, you can check their website (**rtc.li/ca-parks-incidents**) for closure notices.

Wherever you explore, remember to #SharetheTrail (**railstotrails.org/share thetrail**) and #RecreateResponsibly (**recreateresponsibly.org**). Trails continue to welcome more and more people of every age and ability. Together, we can help make every trip safe and fun for everyone.

Key to Trail Use Icons

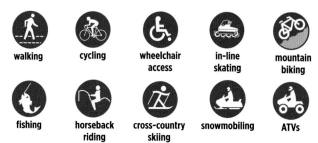

| walking | cycling | wheelchair access | in-line skating | mountain biking |
| fishing | horseback riding | cross-country skiing | snowmobiling | ATVs |

Learn More

To learn about additional multiuse trails in your area or to plan a trip to an area beyond the scope of this book, visit Rails-to-Trails Conservancy's trail-finder website **TrailLink.com,** a free resource with more than 40,000 miles of mapped rail-trails and multiuse trails nationwide.

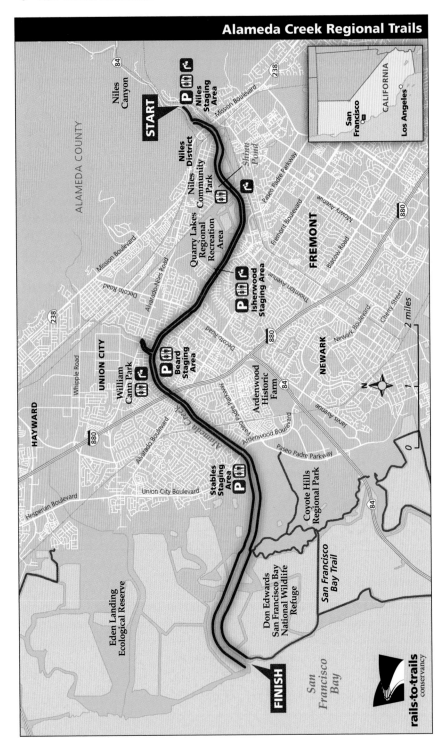

Alameda Creek Regional Trails

The popular Alameda Creek Regional Trails run from the mouth of Niles Canyon in Fremont to the San Francisco Bay, connecting Bay Area neighborhoods with the Indigenous and industrial roots of the region and the rich estuary of the bay.

Featuring northern and southern sections, each roughly 12 miles long, the trails allow recreational access to the levees on both sides of Alameda Creek. The southern section (12 miles), favored by cyclists, is paved until you enter the intertidal zone, where the surface transitions to gravel. The unpaved northern section (12.4 miles) is recommended for equestrians and dog walkers. You'll find access points between the segments at multiple locations along the route. There are also many locations where fishing is permitted in the creek and surrounding ponds, such as Shinn Pond and Quarry Lakes; be sure to verify rules for fishing at each location, as some areas may be protected.

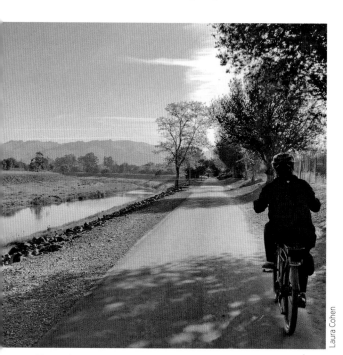

Laura Cohen

The creekside trail runs from the mouth of Niles Canyon to the San Francisco Bay.

County
Alameda

Endpoints
Niles Staging Area on Old Canyon Road, 0.2 mile from Niles Canyon Road (Fremont); San Francisco Bay and Alameda Creek (Fremont)

Mileage
24.4 (12-mile paved southern route; 12.4-mile unpaved northern route)

Type
Greenway/Non-Rail-Trail

Roughness Rating
1–2

Surface
Asphalt, Gravel

The easternmost terminus of the trail is in Fremont, where the Niles District pays homage to the first transcontinental railroad that ran through the region beginning in the late 1800s. On the southern trail segment, accessible parking, restrooms, and a picnic area can be found at the Niles Staging Area, which is dedicated to the brief history of silent movies in the area, which featured stars like Charlie Chaplin. Across the creek, the dog-friendly Niles Community Park is accessible from the northern segment.

As you head west, the trail is dotted with ponds and wildlife as it comes upon the Quarry Lakes Regional Recreation Area, which was formed when gravel was taken for the construction of the western end of the transcontinental railroad. In this densely populated area, the trail also features safe walking and biking connections to the surrounding neighborhoods and transit.

Continuing west, the experience shifts from the wetlands of Alameda Creek to the San Francisco Bay's intertidal zone. This area between high and low tide is an important habitat for many bird and wildlife species and is a haven for

The scenic east–west route traverses Fremont in the East Bay region.   Danielle Casavant

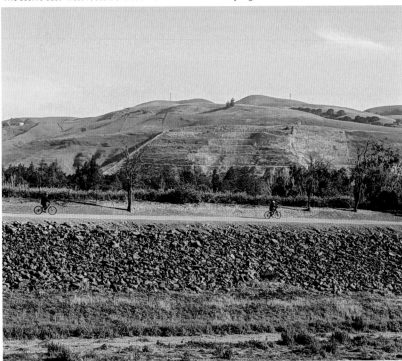

birders. Picnic areas and benches dot the trail. In some locations, bike racks are located adjacent to walking paths into the surrounding wetlands. Bird species that may be found along the trail include the pied-billed grebe, northern shoveler, great blue heron, spotted sandpiper, American coot, and white pelican. As the trail approaches the San Francisco Bay, the freshwater of Alameda Creek and the saltwater of the Pacific mix, forming an estuary that's home to many native fish and bird species and serves as a natural barrier controlling floods, erosion, pollution, and sediment. The westernmost regional park along the trail is Coyote Hills, 1,266 acres of marshland and rolling hills where visitors come to walk, jog, bicycle, bird-watch, and picnic on the ancestral homeland of the Tuibun Ohlone peoples, who originally settled the area and relied on the creek as a resource. (Programming about the area's Indigenous history is available in the park.)

A portion of the Alameda Creek Regional Trails is also a significant component of the San Francisco Bay Trail, a developing effort to create a 500-mile multiuse trail encircling its namesake bay. Both are part of the developing 2,590-mile Bay Area regional trail network being spearheaded by the Bay Area Trails Collaborative (**railstotrails.org/bay-area**) and Rails-to-Trails Conservancy as a TrailNation™ project to increase safe walking, biking, and trail access for millions of Bay Area residents.

Closure Notice: Due to the 2022–2023 storms, three underpasses along the Alameda Creek Regional Trails are closed and inaccessible to the public until further notice. Visit the website below for details.

CONTACT rtc.li/alameda-creek

PARKING

Parking locations are listed from east to west. *Indicates that at least one accessible parking space is available.*

FREMONT* Niles Staging Area, Old Canyon Road, 0.2 mile from Niles Canyon Road (37.5794, -121.9660).

FREMONT* Isherwood Staging Area, Isherwood Way, 370 feet north of Paseo Padre Pkwy. (37.5723, -122.0131).

FREMONT* Beard Staging Area, Beard Road, 375 feet north of Sanderling Dr./Whitehead Lane (37.5873, -122.0393).

UNION CITY* Stables Staging Area, Eastin Dr. at Eastin Ct., 200 feet south of Union City Blvd. (37.5646, -122.0702).

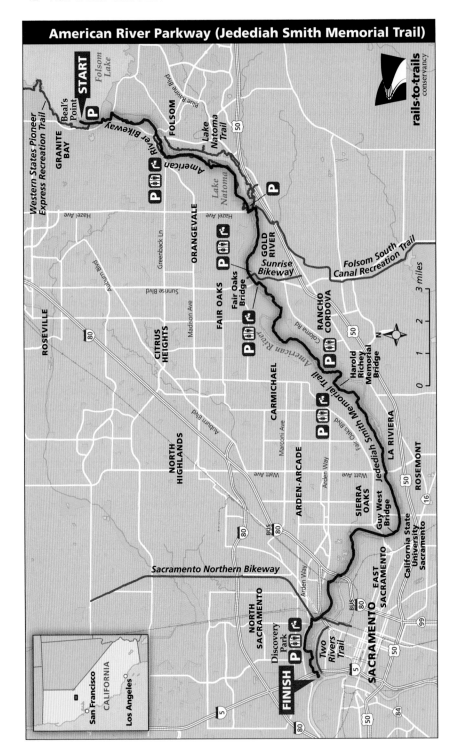

American River Parkway (Jedediah Smith Memorial Trail)

rails·to·trails
conservancy

This Northern California pathway follows the American River as it flows through riparian habitat preserved by the American River Parkway. The scenic trail runs for 32 miles between Folsom Lake's southwestern banks at Beal's Point and Discovery Park in Old Town Sacramento.

For the easiest bike ride, you can start at the northeast end of the trail at Beal's Point and travel downhill. The first 8.4 miles of the trail are managed by California State Parks; here, signage refers to the trail as the American River Bikeway. Beginning at Hazel Avenue, the trail is signed as the Jedediah Smith Memorial Trail and is managed by Sacramento County.

The two-lane trail is fully paved, with mile markers, trailside maps, water fountains, and restrooms along the way. Note that signage advises walkers and runners to

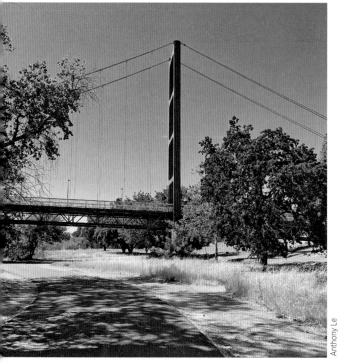

The Guy West Bridge provides access to the California State University, Sacramento, campus.

Anthony Le

County
Sacramento

Endpoints
Beal's Point and Oak Hill Dr. (Granite Bay); Jibboom St. and Natomas Park Dr. in Discovery Park (Sacramento)

Mileage
32

Type
Greenway/Non-Rail-Trail

Roughness Rating
1

Surface
Asphalt

stay on the left side or shoulder of the trail; stay alert while passing. The trail provides picturesque views of Folsom Lake, Lake Natoma, and the American River. It connects with a number of other trails, including the Western States Pioneer Express Recreation Trail, Lake Natoma Trail (see page 117), Folsom South Canal Recreation Trail, Sunrise Bikeway, Sacramento Northern Bikeway (see page 191), and Two Rivers Trail. Multiple unpaved hiking trails also intersect it.

Many beautiful pedestrian bridges cross the river along the route: the Fair Oaks Bridge, a truss bridge built in the early 1900s; the Harold Richey Memorial Bridge, which connects River Bend Park to the William B. Pond Recreation Area; and the Guy West Bridge, a suspension bridge that links the trail to the California State University, Sacramento, campus.

The trail is mostly level, although the route does traverse some rolling terrain. About half the route is shaded by trees, while the other half offers views of wildflower fields. Along the way, you'll pass through several parks and swimming areas, as well as the suburban enclaves of Sacramento.

Caution: Due to the 2022–2023 storms, flooding damage can be found in areas along the west end of the American River Parkway from Discovery Park to Watt Avenue. Visit Sacramento County's regional parks web page for details: **rtc.li/saccounty.**

CONTACT arpf.org

PARKING

Parking areas are listed from north to south. Select parking areas for the trail are listed below. For a detailed list of parking areas and other waypoints, go to **TrailLink.com**™. *Indicates that at least one accessible parking space is available.*

GRANITE BAY* Beal's Point, 275 feet east of Oak Hill Dr. (38.7206, -121.1686); parking fee.

FOLSOM* Black Miners Bar on Park Road, 0.2 mile south of Greenback Lane (38.6804, -121.1848).

GOLD RIVER* Sacramento State Aquatic Center, 1901 Hazel Ave. (38.6342, -121.2208).

RANCHO CORDOVA* Upper Sunrise Boat Ramp on S. Bridge St., 0.8 mile northeast of Sunrise Blvd. (38.6357, -121.2641).

RANCHO CORDOVA* Sunrise Recreation Area on S. Bridge St., 0.3 mile west of Sunrise Blvd. (38.6318, -121.2699).

RANCHO CORDOVA* Hagan Community Park, 2197 Chase Dr. (38.6041, -121.3102).

CARMICHAEL* William B. Pond Recreation Area on Arden Way, 0.3 mile from McClaren Dr. (38.5880, -121.3351).

SACRAMENTO* Discovery Park on Natomas Park Dr., 0.7 mile southwest of Garden Hwy. (38.6003, -121.5080).

Located on the eastern edge of the San Francisco Bay Area, the Arroyo Mocho Trail is a tale of two trails. From its western starting point at West Las Positas Boulevard in Pleasanton to near El Charro Road (about 5 miles), its surface is loose gravel interspersed with some brief paved areas. If cycling, wide tires and experience on loose gravel are recommended. This section is quite suitable for walking and jogging but is not wheelchair or road-bike friendly. The trail runs mostly below street level here and follows the Arroyo Mocho. A paralleling upper trail allows access to the surrounding neighborhoods and nearby Ken Mercer Sports Park. East of El Charro Road, the trail runs alongside major roadways but is separated from them and feels safe from traffic. The first 9 miles of trail offer little to no shade cover or easily accessible water, so plan ahead on hot days.

County
Alameda

Endpoints
Centennial Trail, 0.2 mile south of W. Las Positas Blvd. (Pleasanton); Stanley Blvd. and Isabel Ave. (Livermore); Concannon Blvd. and Normandy Cir. (Livermore); Sunken Gardens Skate Park (Livermore); Almond Ave., between Blossom Cir. and Almond Cir. (Livermore); Charlotte Way and Stockton Loop (Livermore)

Mileage
12.9

Type
Greenway/Non-Rail-Trail

Roughness Rating
1–2

Surface
Asphalt, Concrete, Gravel

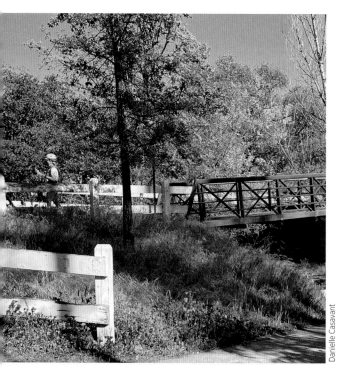

Danielle Casavant

Approaching Livermore, the trail meanders through several parks and natural areas.

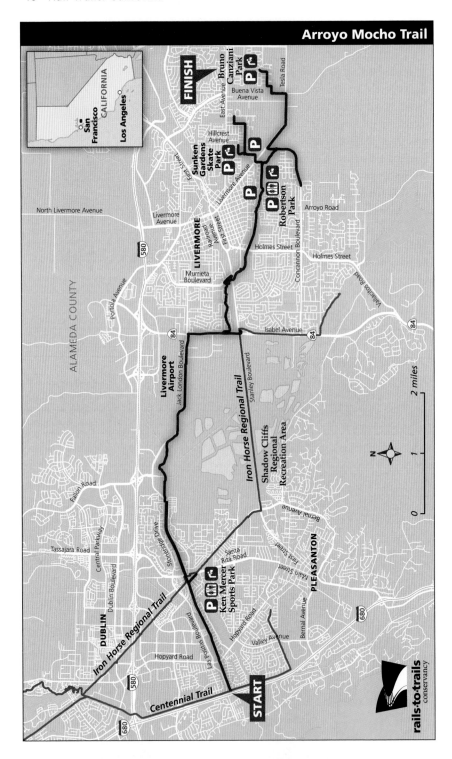

Arroyo Mocho Trail

As the trail approaches Livermore, it transitions to a more neighborhood feel. The Livermore area is home to many wineries and a brewery not far from the trail. This portion also has many direct access points from the surrounding neighborhoods, which are filled with citrus trees and grapevines that make for an inviting backdrop. For 2.2 miles, the trail meanders through several parks and natural areas with more shade available. There is an equestrian arena at Robertson Park, as well as restrooms and water.

Just east of Robertson Park, the trail branches both north and south. The north branch takes you around Sunken Gardens Skate Park (aka Livermore Skate Park) and ends in a residential area at Almond Avenue. The skate park offers parking and drinking fountains but no restrooms. The south branch of the trail continues 0.4 mile before splitting at Concannon Boulevard: The northeastern route heads toward Bruno Canziani Park, which has parking, drinking fountains, a dog park, and children's play equipment but no restrooms. The southwest branch takes you along Concannon Boulevard to Normandy Circle. You'll travel through a vineyard area with a winery adjacent to the trail.

CONTACT larpd.org/trails

PARKING

Parking locations are listed from west to east. **Indicates that at least one accessible parking space is available.*

PLEASANTON* Ken Mercer Sports Park, 5800 Parkside Dr. (37.6810, -121.8945).

LIVERMORE Robertson Park on Robertson Park Road, 0.3 mile east of Arroyo Road (37.6708, -121.7628).

LIVERMORE Robertson Park on Robertson Park Road, 0.5 mile west of Concannon Blvd. (37.6690, -121.7565).

LIVERMORE* Sunken Gardens Skate Park, 3800 Pacific Ave. (37.6757, -121.7508).

LIVERMORE* Robertson Park Disc Golf Course, 1505 S. Livermore Ave. (37.6703, -121.7509).

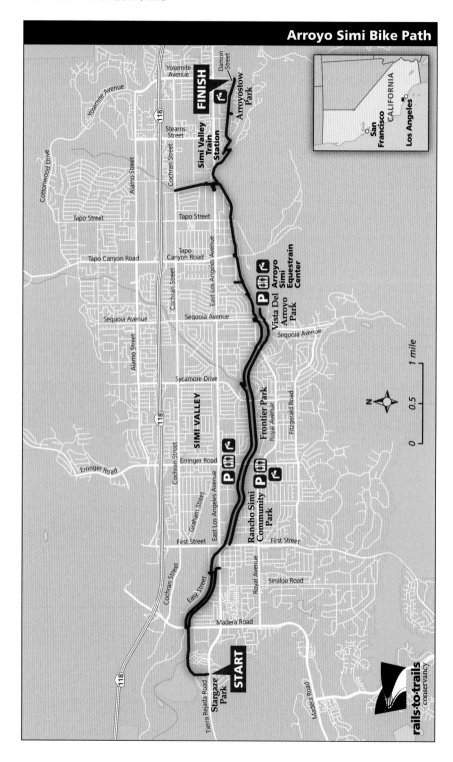

Arroyo Simi Bike Path

CALIFORNIA

San Francisco

Los Angeles

Yosemite Avenue

Damon Street

Yosemite Avenue

FINISH

Arroyostow Park

118

Stearns Street

Simi Valley Train Station

Cottonwood Drive

Alamo Street

Cochran Street

Tapo Street

Tapo Street

Tapo Canyon Road

Tapo Canyon Road

East Los Angeles Avenue

Cochran Street

Vista Del Arroyo Park

P

Arroyo Simi Equestrain Center

Sequoia Avenue

Sequoia Avenue

Sequoia Avenue

Alamo Street

Sycamore Drive

SIMI VALLEY

N

Frontier Park

Royal Avenue

Fitzgerald Road

1 mile

0.5

0

Cochran Street

Erringer Road

Erringer Road

P

Rancho Simi Community Park

P

118

Graham Street

East Los Angeles Avenue

First Street

First Street

Royal Avenue

Sinaloa Road

Easy Street

Madera Road

Cochran Street

118

START

Stargaze Park

Tierra Rejada Road

Royal Avenue

Madera Road

rails-to-trails conservancy

The 8.6-mile Arroyo Simi Bike Path traverses Simi Valley in Ventura County. The majority of this rail-with-trail follows the Arroyo Simi, the creek for which the trail is named, and which serves as a flood-control channel. The trail runs along both the northern and southern sides of the creek for much of the trail. Multiple bridges allow users to switch between the northern and southern sides.

To follow the southern side, begin at Tierra Rejada Road and Stargaze Place. From here, users will enjoy a short on-road segment within a residential neighborhood featuring lovely landscaping, flowers, and a soft surface. The surface quickly changes to paved as the trail transitions to a greenway heading up a somewhat steep hill with scenic views. Users with accessibility needs may want to skip this part of the journey and start at Madera Road, 0.8 mile east of the western endpoint. Madera Road is also the first point at which you can access the trail's northern side.

County
Ventura

Endpoints
Southern: Tierra Rejada Road and Stargaze Pl. (Simi Valley); Los Angeles Ave. and Fifth St. (Simi Valley); First St., just north of Pacific Ave. (Simi Valley); Chicory Leaf Pl., 0.2 mile from Sequoia Ave. (Simi Valley) *Northern:* Madera Road, between E. Easy St. and Aristotle St. (Simi Valley); Cochran St., between Fig St. and Ralston St. (Simi Valley); Yosemite Ave., just south of Damon St. (Simi Valley)

Mileage
8.6

Type
Greenway/Non-Rail-Trail, Rail-with-Trail

Roughness Rating
1

Surface
Asphalt, Crushed Stone

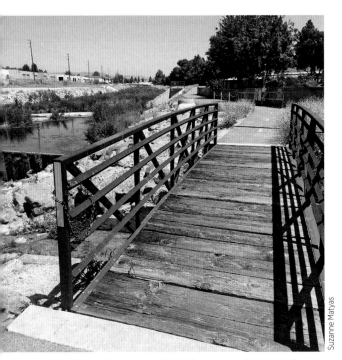

The neighborhood trail traverses Simi Valley in the greater Los Angeles area.

The trail continues over a footbridge and then takes its typical formation along the Arroyo Simi. This main part of the trail includes some minor hills, dips, and bumpy sections that could be challenging for wheelchairs. In addition, many of the street access points and crossings are heavily trafficked and lack on-street bicycle infrastructure.

For most of the journey, the trail sits above the Arroyo Simi. Near East Los Angeles Avenue, however, the trail goes beneath an on-street bridge and brings users down closer to the creek. Be on the lookout for turkey vultures, hawks, greater yellowlegs, belted kingfishers, killdeers, common yellowthroats, American kestrels, and ducks.

A highlight of the trail is the beautiful Rancho Simi Community Park, which includes sports facilities, water fountains, restrooms, and the tree-rimmed Rancho Simi Park Lake, a popular local duck pond and fishing hole. About a half-mile farther down the trail, you will arrive at the much smaller Frontier Park, which boasts a historical cannon and playground equipment. The portion of trail following the southern side of the creek ends at Vista Del Arroyo Park, a modern facility with a playground, a gazebo with a picnic table, and a basketball court. Adjacent to the park is the Arroyo Simi Equestrian Center. Horseback riding, while permitted on the trail, is more popular on the regional trails around the equestrian center, especially heading east from here.

The portion of trail following the northern side of the creek continues past the Simi Valley rail station, where Metrolink's Ventura County Line and Amtrak are both available. You may even catch a glimpse of a train on this rail-with-trail segment. Near the end of the trail, you will find the grassy Arroyostow Park, which offers mountain views and play equipment. The trail ends at Yosemite Avenue near Damon Street.

CONTACT rtc.li/arroyo-simi-bikepath

PARKING

Parking areas are located within Simi Valley and are listed from west to east. *Indicates that at least one accessible parking space is available.

RANCHO SIMI COMMUNITY PARK, WEST RESTROOM* Thompson Lane and Royal Ave. (34.2664, -118.7661).

RANCHO SIMI COMMUNITY PARK, EAST RESTROOM* Erringer Road, across from Elizondo Ave. (34.2657, -118.7616).

ARROYO SIMI EQUESTRIAN CENTER Chicory Leaf Pl. (34.2636, -118.7279); horse trailer parking available.

SIMI VALLEY AMTRAK STATION* 5050 E. Los Angeles Ave. (34.2706, -118.6955).

The Ballona Creek Bike Path follows Ballona Creek along its meandering banks through the residential neighborhoods of western Los Angeles. Beginning at the mouth of the creek overlooking the Pacific Ocean and ending in bustling downtown Culver City, this trail provides users with a unique recreational experience that combines an exploration of the iconic concrete channels of Los Angeles' watershed with unparalleled opportunities for wildflower viewing and bird-watching.

At its western end, the Ballona Creek Bike Path connects to the Marvin Braude Bike Trail (see page 133), a 22-mile trail that travels along Los Angeles' coastline. You can take that trail to catch a glimpse of whales, dolphins, and sea lions frolicking in the Pacific Ocean, or explore the nearby neighborhoods of Venice Beach, Marina del Rey, and Playa del Rey. The western end of the Ballona Creek trail is also your best opportunity to view waterfowl

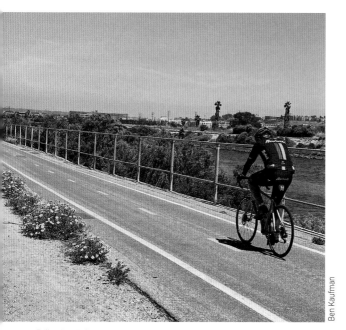

Following Ballona Creek, the path meanders through the neighborhoods of western Los Angeles.

Ben Kaufman

County
Los Angeles

Endpoints
Marvin Braude Bike Trail adjacent to Ballona Creek, 0.1 mile southeast of Fiji Way (Marina del Rey); southeast corner of Syd Kronenthal Park at the Exposition Line Bikeway (Culver City)

Mileage
6.4

Type
Greenway/Non-Rail-Trail

Roughness Rating
1

Surface
Asphalt, Concrete

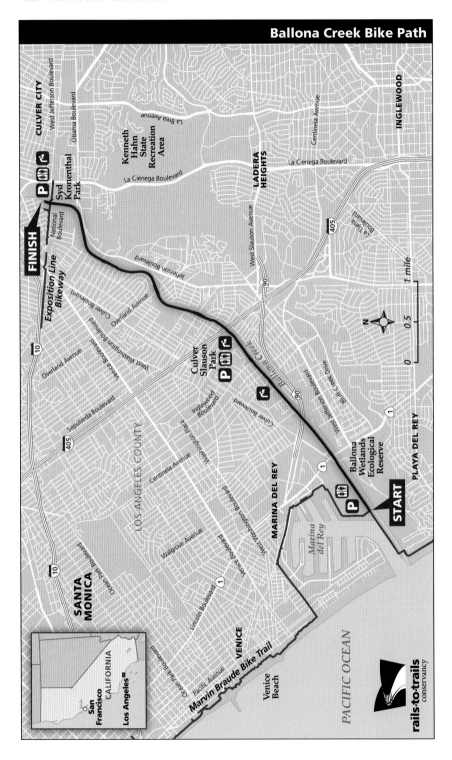

Ballona Creek Bike Path

in the Ballona Wetlands Ecological Reserve, the last remaining wetlands habitat in Los Angeles. Keep your eyes peeled for herons, egrets, godwits, pelicans, cormorants, and ospreys, among other wetlands species.

At its eastern end, the trail connects to the Exposition Line Bikeway, which travels through downtown Culver City and follows the Los Angeles Metro E Line light rail (formerly the Expo Line) west to downtown Santa Monica. Exit the trail at Syd Kronenthal Park to observe a pick-up baseball game, grab a bite to eat at one of the streetside cafés along hip and historic Culver Boulevard, or hop on the E Line and enjoy a relaxing ride to a completely different part of LA.

If you plan to travel the whole trail in one fell swoop, be sure to use the restroom and stock up on water and other provisions beforehand, as there are few restrooms or concessions along the trail. That said, the trail is well-connected to the LA street grid, so there are ample opportunities to peel off and find a local coffee shop or grocery store to restock. The endpoints of the trail are your best bet, although there are several streets along the way that may also have what you're looking for, including Centinela Avenue, Sepulveda Boulevard, and Obama Boulevard.

Along the Ballona Creek Bike Path, there are several paid parking lots at both ends of the trail, as well as parking opportunities in adjacent parks and ample street parking throughout the neighborhoods in between. Water fountains, seating areas, and shade structures can be found sporadically throughout the trail, becoming most prevalent on the eastern end of the trail, east of I-405.

CONTACT trails.lacounty.gov/trail/91/ballona-creek-bike-path

PARKING

Parking areas are listed from west to east. *Indicates that at least one accessible parking space is available.*

MARINA DEL REY* 13745 Fiji Way (33.9731, -118.4459); parking fees may apply.

LOS ANGELES* Culver Slauson Park, 5070 S. Slauson Ave. (33.9937, -118.4066).

CULVER CITY* Syd Kronenthal Park, 3459 McManus Ave. (34.0280, -118.3774).

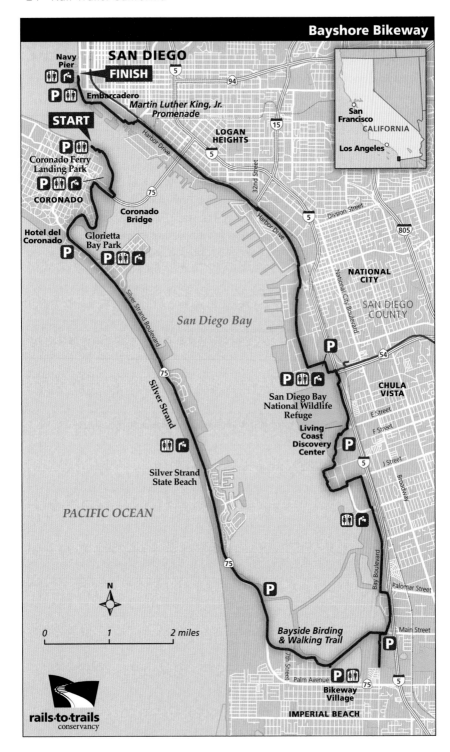

Bayshore Bikeway

Nearly encircling the San Diego Bay, the Bayshore Bikeway offers views of downtown San Diego and the resort town of Coronado while providing access to a number of parks and beaches. Currently, the 24-mile route includes 17.1 miles of completed multiuse pathway, with the rest consisting of on-road sections. The pathway is also a segment of the California Coastal Trail, a network of bicycling and hiking trails that, when complete, will stretch along the coastline for 1,230 miles from Oregon to the Mexican border.

Since much of the route on the eastern side of the bay entails on-road riding, exploring the western side makes for an easier, more relaxing experience. Note that there is no shade along the trail, so be sure to wear sun protection and bring water.

The route begins at Coronado Ferry Landing Park on the northern tip of the Bayshore Bikeway, where parking, restrooms, bike rental shops, and restaurants are readily available. Within minutes of setting off, you'll be treated to a spectacular vista of the Coronado Bridge, which

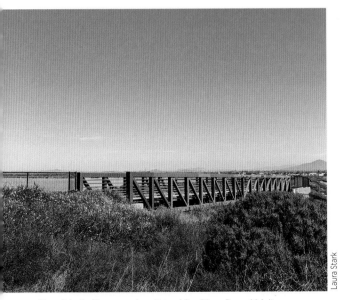

The rail-trail offers sweeping views of San Diego Bay, which it nearly encircles.

Laura Stark

County
San Diego

Endpoints
Coronado Ferry Landing Park, at First St. and B Ave. (Coronado); Navy Pier and N. Harbor Dr. (San Diego)

Mileage
17.1

Type
Rail-Trail

Roughness Rating
1

Surface
Asphalt, Concrete

received an Award of Merit in the American Institute of Steel Construction's 1970 selection of the country's most beautiful bridges open to traffic, and—in true California style—you'll hit your first beach in less than a mile. You'll also pass by the iconic Hotel del Coronado, which was built in 1888 and has been the backdrop for a few movies, including Marilyn Monroe's *Some Like It Hot.*

Continuing south from the hotel, the pathway follows the Silver Strand, the narrow spit of land that separates San Diego Bay from the Pacific Ocean and on which the Coronado branch of the San Diego and Arizona Eastern Railway once traveled. Construction of the railroad began under prominent San Diego resident John D. Spreckels in 1906 and was completed in 1919.

On the left, you'll find Glorietta Bay Park, which offers a beach, a playground, a picnic area, and restrooms. Although the rail-trail parallels CA 75 on this stretch, wildflowers and brush along the route keep the journey pleasant as you continue south.

As you approach the south end of the bay, you'll have spacious views of the San Diego Bay National Wildlife Refuge. Its preserved wetlands offer prime opportunities for birding and support many endangered and threatened species of flora and fauna. As you enter the residential community of Imperial Beach, look for the entrance to the Bayside Birding & Walking Trail at Seventh Street; the dirt pathway parallels the Bayshore Bikeway for 0.4 mile and has interpretive panels on topics like migratory birds and salt marsh restoration.

On the bikeway's north end, enjoy a spectacular vista of the Coronado Bridge.   Laura Stark

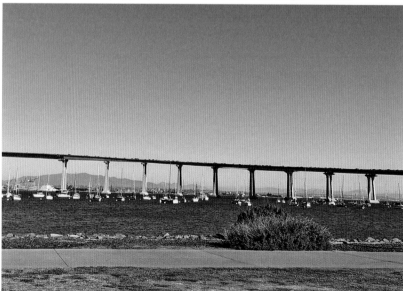

After continuing east 0.8 mile from the entrance to the birding trail, take the opportunity to turn right at the short trail spur just before the red pedestrian bridge to reach Imperial Beach's Bikeway Village, where you'll find public restrooms and a coffee shop where you can pick up snacks and refreshments. The continuous, paved portion of the rail-trail ends 1 mile farther on at Main Street and West Frontage Road in Chula Vista.

If you would like to continue on the Bayshore Bikeway along the east side of the bay, follow the marked on-road bike lanes (largely paralleling Bay Boulevard) and a few short stretches of paved pathway north through Chula Vista and into San Diego. A highlight of this section is Chula Vista's Living Coast Discovery Center, which features interactive exhibits on the animals and plants of coastal California. As you approach the Coronado Bridge, be sure to also check out the colorful collection of murals in Chicano Park, which celebrates the heritage and culture of Barrio Logan, San Diego's oldest Mexican-American neighborhood.

Note that the bikeway is currently under construction at South 32nd Street and Harbor Drive. Until this segment is completed in 2025, follow the signed alternative route to close a 2.5-mile gap to Park Boulevard. From there, the trail picks up again at the Embarcadero, San Diego's popular waterfront pathway, and ends at the Navy Pier and USS Midway Museum (housed in a historical naval aircraft carrier).

CONTACT rtc.li/bayshore-bway

PARKING

Parking areas are listed counterclockwise from the Coronado end of the Bayshore Bikeway to the San Diego end. Select parking areas for the trail are listed below. For a detailed list of parking areas and other waypoints, go to **TrailLink.com**™. *Indicates that at least one accessible parking space is available.*

CORONADO* Coronado Ferry Landing, 1201 First St. (32.6982, -117.1692); nominal parking fee.

CORONADO* Coronado Tidelands Park, 2000 Mullinex Dr. (32.6913, -117.1652).

CORONADO* Glorietta Bay Park, 1975 Strand Way (32.6753, -117.1696).

IMPERIAL BEACH* Bayshore Bikeway Parking Lot; accessible only from northbound CA 75, 1.3 mile north of Seventh St. (32.6023, -117.1241).

IMPERIAL BEACH* Biking Village, 13th Street and Cypress Ave. (32.5874, -117.1057).

CHULA VISTA* Bay Boulevard Park, F St. and Bay Blvd. (32.6359, -117.0999).

NATIONAL CITY* Pepper Park, 3299 Tidelands Ave. (32.6503, -117.1114).

SAN DIEGO* Embarcadero Marina Park North, 400 Kettner Blvd. (32.7074, -117.1694); nominal parking fee.

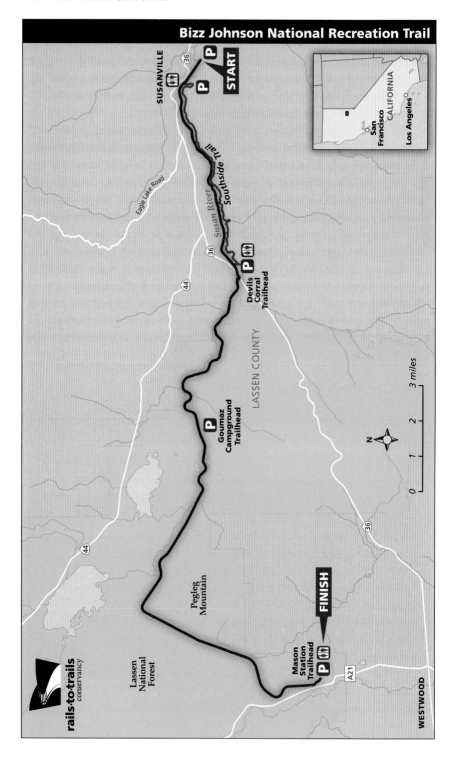

An outing on the Bizz Johnson National Recreation Trail rewards trekkers with eye-catching Northern California scenery and signs of wildlife. The 25.4-mile packed gravel-and-dirt trail connects the historical logging towns of Susanville and Westwood on a remote route that passes through tunnels and crosses the Susan River on numerous bridges.

Known simply as The Bizz, the rail-trail follows the route of the old Fernley and Lassen Railway line, which was established in 1914 to haul logs and milled lumber between a mill in Westwood and the Southern Pacific Railroad's main line at Fernley, Nevada. The mill closed in 1956, and the railroad ceased operations in 1978. The Bureau of Land Management and former US Representative Harold T. "Bizz" Johnson, who represented the district in Congress from 1958 to 1980, spearheaded the

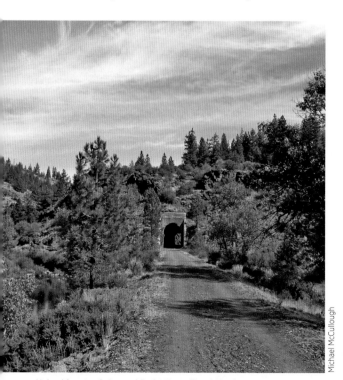

Upland forests of pine and fir dot the trail's arid landscape.

Michael McCullough

County
Lassen

Endpoints
Susanville Depot (Susanville); Mason Station (Westwood)

Mileage
25.4

Type
Rail-Trail

Roughness Rating
2

Surface
Dirt, Gravel

conversion of the corridor into a rail-trail. The pathway—listed in Rails-to-Trails Conservancy's Hall of Fame—is named in his honor.

Before setting out, visitors can view exhibits at the Lassen Land and Trails Trust, which is housed in a 1927 vintage railroad depot in Susanville. The trail starts at a caboose across the street and begins a gentle climb along the rushing Susan River. The eastern 7 miles are the most popular, as the trail passes through a semiarid, rocky canyon where the compacted surface is wheelchair accessible. For those who wish to take a slightly different route, the singletrack Southside Trail traces the south bank of the river through the canyon.

Trees on the riverbank make this a colorful journey in the fall, and travelers will cross several bridges and pass through two tunnels in the canyon. Jumbles of sticks and earthen mounds along the river mark beaver and muskrat dams and lodges, and sharp-eyed visitors might see raccoons, mule deer, porcupines, and coyotes at dawn or dusk. More than 100 bird species have been documented here.

The trail emerges from the canyon at the Devils Corral trailhead on CA 36. Leaving the Great Basin Desert habitat behind, it enters the pine and fir forests of the Sierra Nevada and Cascade ranges. The 9,000-acre Hog Fire that swept the area in 2020 left scorched patches in this once dense woodland.

The trail continues climbing for another 10.4 miles to the foot of Pegleg Mountain, where it leaves the Susan River and begins a slight downhill grade for

The trail follows the old Fernley and Lassen Railway route.   Michael McCullough

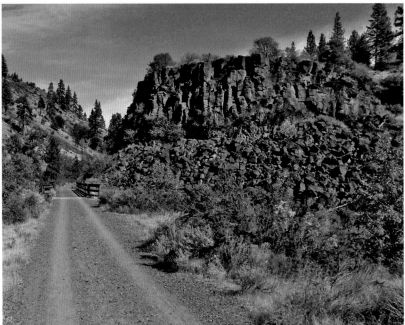

7.6 miles to end at Mason Station Trailhead. From here it's another 4.5 miles along McCoy Road and Mooney Road/A21 to the nearest town, Westwood. Here you'll find a museum and replica of the Westwood Depot, as well as a 25-foot redwood carving of Paul Bunyan. The Lassen Rural Bus provides bike-rack-equipped bus service between Westwood and Susanville (**lassentransportation.com**). When visiting, remember there are no services between Susanville and Westwood. Spring and fall weather can be fickle, as the trail elevations range from 4,100 to 5,500 feet. The U.S. Forest Service, which manages the 18 trail miles west of Devils Corral, allows snowmobiling when winter conditions permit. Primitive camping is allowed throughout.

Those who visit the Saturday of Columbus Day weekend will enjoy the Lassen Land and Trails Trust's annual Rails to Trails Festival in Susanville. The festival, which raises funds to support the region's trails, includes live music, a chili cook-off, handcar races, and other fun family activities.

CONTACT blm.gov/visit/bizz-johnson and lassenlandandtrailstrust.org

PARKING

Parking areas are listed from east to west. *Indicates that at least one accessible parking space is available.*

SUSANVILLE* Susanville Depot, 601 Richmond Road (40.4117, -120.6602).

SUSANVILLE* Bizz Johnson Trail Susanville Trailhead, 514 Richmond Road (40.411502, -120.6608).

SUSANVILLE* Hobo Camp Trailhead, at the end of Hobo Camp Road, 0.7 mile northwest of South St. (40.4174, -120.6736).

SUSANVILLE* Devils Corral Trailhead, CA 36/Volcanic Legacy Scenic Byway, 1.6 miles southeast of CA 44/Feather Lake Hwy. (40.3981, -120.7737).

SUSANVILLE* Goumaz Campground Trailhead, Forest Road 30N03, 3 miles south of CA 44 (40.4139, -120.8619).

WESTWOOD* Mason Station Trailhead, McCoy Road, 0.4 mile north of the intersection of McCoy and Mooney Roads (40.3621, -120.9992).

Browns Creek Bike Path and Orange Line Bike Path

CALIFORNIA

San Francisco

Los Angeles

Coldwater Canyon Avenue

FINISH

Woodman Avenue

Sherman Way

Vanowen Street

Victory Boulevard

Oxnard Street

Burbank Boulevard

Magnolia Boulevard

VAN NUYS

Van Nuys Avenue

Roscoe Boulevard

Nordhoff Street

Parthenia Street

Saticoy Street

Van Nuys Avenue

Kester Avenue

SHERMAN OAKS

Sepulveda Boulevard

405

405

Woodley Avenue

Woodley Avenue

Sepulveda Basin Recreation Area

Hayvenhurts Avenue

Van Nuys Airport

ENCINO

101

2 miles

Balboa Boulevard

P

P

Saticoy Street

RESEDA

White Oak Avenue

LOS ANGELES COUNTY

NORTHRIDGE

N

1

0

Reseda Boulevard

Victory Boulevard

Oxnard Street

Ventura Boulevard

Nordhoff Street

Parthenia Street

Wilbur Avenue

Sherman Way

Vanowen Street

Orange Line Bike Path

Tampa Avenue

WINNETKA

TARZANA

101

Corbin Avenue

Los Angeles River Greenway

Lassen Street

Plummer Street

Devonshire Street

START

Roscoe Boulevard

Parthenia Street

Winnetka Avenue

Mason Avenue

CHATSWORTH

CANOGA PARK

Saticoy Street

De Soto Avenue

Canoga Avenue

Browns Creek Bike Path

Orange Line Bike Path

WOODLAND HILLS

Topanga Canyon Boulevard

Sherman Way

Vanowen Street

rails-to-trails conservancy

Enjoy a 17-mile trek across multiple Los Angeles neighborhoods on this former Southern Pacific Railroad corridor. The Orange Line Bike Path follows the G Line (formerly Orange Line) rapid bus route's dedicated corridor, meaning LA traffic is not a concern here. With bus stations and bike lockers along the route of the trail, traveling by a combination of bike and bus is a breeze. The buses all have bike racks, so you can bike the entire route, put your bike on the bus, and take it back to where you started.

The trail traverses dense neighborhoods, heavily trafficked roads, and light industrial areas. What it lacks in beauty, however, it makes up for in functionality. There are many heavily trafficked at-grade road crossings that will take some patience to cross, but they are all signalized.

For the longest on-trail journey possible, start at North Independence Avenue and Rinaldi Street, the northern endpoint of the 1.5-mile Browns Creek Bike

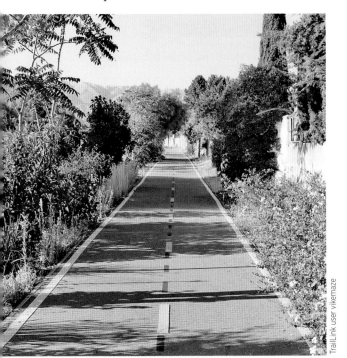

Browns Creek Bike Path traverses the Chatsworth neighborhood.

TrailLink user vikemaze

County
Los Angeles

Endpoints
N. Independence Ave. and Rinaldi St. (Los Angeles); Leghorn Ave. and Chandler Blvd. (Los Angeles)

Mileage
17.3

Type
Rail-Trail (Orange Line Bike Path)/ Greenway/ Non-Rail-Trail (Browns Creek Bike Path)

Roughness Rating
1

Surface
Asphalt, Concrete

Path. This segment includes some murals and pleasant vegetation running along a channelized waterway. As you go farther south, the trail abuts warehouses. Following a short, one-block gap at Lassen Street, you will officially find yourself on the Orange Line Bike Path.

In about 3.75 miles, the trail crosses over a segment of the developing 51-mile Los Angeles River Greenway (also known as the Los Angeles River Trail) just north of the intersection of Canoga Avenue and Vanowen Street, but unfortunately there is not a safe way for bicyclists or pedestrians to connect to it here from the Orange Line Bike Path. The trail will then lead you east to the sprawling Sepulveda Basin Recreation Area, which includes a lake, boat and bike rentals, a Japanese garden, an archery range, a model aircraft field, a golf course, sports fields, parking, and restrooms. You can access an additional segment of the Los Angeles River Greenway just past the park's southeast border in the Sepulveda Basin Recreation Area at Sepulveda Boulevard and Valleyheart Drive.

Continuing east from the park is a wide, tree-lined segment, followed by a unique portion where the trail weaves beneath the elevated infrastructure of I-405. The route then takes you away from the street for some much-needed peace and quiet.

The trail ends at Chandler Boulevard and Leghorn Avenue. From here, an unprotected bike lane connects to the 2.8-mile Chandler Bikeway, heading east. Plans are in the works to connect these trails via an approximately 3-mile separated cycle track.

CONTACT laparks.org/info/biking and **metro.net/projects/orangeline**

PARKING

Parking areas are located within Los Angeles and are listed from north to south. *Indicates that at least one accessible parking space is available.*

SEPULVEDA BASIN SPORTS COMPLEX* 6301 Balboa Blvd. (34.1840, -118.5020).

SEPULVEDA BASIN SPORTS COMPLEX* Balboa Blvd., 0.6 mile south of Victory Blvd. (34.1790, -118.5015).

The Cal Park Hill Tunnel and SMART Pathway are located in the heart of the Marin County suburbs, spanning 2.5 miles between Larkspur and San Rafael. This convenient rail-with-trail is perfect for commuting, as it cuts underneath the 200-foot Cal Park Hill and runs adjacent to the Sonoma–Marin Area Rail Transit (SMART) commuter train. Additionally, the southern end of the trail is just steps from the Larkspur Ferry Terminal, which provides direct service to downtown San Francisco. Along the way, there are plenty of wayfinding signs, maps, and trailside markers to guide you, and the smooth, paved surface provides an accessible transportation route for all types of trail users.

Although the trail is relatively short, it's part of a planned 70-mile SMART Pathway system that will eventually connect Marin and Sonoma Counties from Larkspur

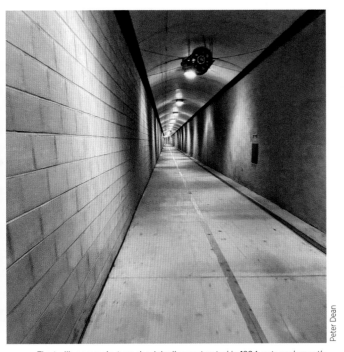

The trail's namesake tunnel, originally constructed in 1884, cuts underneath the 200-foot Cal Park Hill.

Peter Dean

County
Marin

Endpoints
Sir Francis Drake Blvd. and Redwood Hwy./ US 101 (Larkspur); Second St. and Francisco Blvd. W. (San Rafael)

Mileage
2.5

Type
Rail-with-Trail

Roughness Rating
1

Surface
Asphalt, Concrete

Cal Park Hill Tunnel and SMART Pathway

3rd Street

San Rafael
SMART Station

Second Street

FINISH

Lincoln Avenue

Francisco Boulevard West

3rd Street

San Rafael Creek

San Francisco

CALIFORNIA

Los Angeles

Irwin Street

Rice Drive

101

Andersen Drive

Francisco Boulevard West

Francisco Boulevard East

Belvedere Street

Kerner Boulevard

SAN RAFAEL

SMART Pathway

Irwin Street

Woodland Avenue

Woodland Avenue

Bellam Boulevard

Bellam Boulevard

MARIN COUNTY

N

580

Jacoby Street

Andersen Drive

0   0.25   0.5 mile

101

Redwood Highway

Cal Park
Hill Tunnel

LARKSPUR

Sir Francis Drake Boulevard

Larkspur
SMART
Station

Larkspur
Landing
Shopping
Center

Larkspur
Landing
Circle

San Francisco Bay Trail

Sir Francis Drake Boulevard

Larkspur
Ferry
Terminal

START

Corte Madera Creek

101

North-South
Greenway

Redwood Highway

rails·to·trails
conservancy

to Cloverdale. Currently, 24 miles of the pathway are completed, with another 14.5 funded or under construction. The SMART Pathway is also part of a developing 2,600-miles-plus Bay Area regional trail network being spearheaded by the Bay Area Trails Collaborative (**railstotrails.org/bay-area**) and Rails-to-Trails Conservancy as a TrailNation™ project to increase safe walking, biking, and trail access for millions of Bay Area residents.

From the trail's southern endpoint, you'll take a ramp up to a pedestrian bridge over Sir Francis Drake Boulevard and reach SMART's Larkspur station in 0.2 mile. Although the trail is situated in a dense urban area, as you continue north you'll be safely separated from road traffic and separated by a fence from the commuter train. Pockets of trees provide welcome shade.

From the SMART station, it's another 0.3 mile to the trail's highlight: the Cal Park Hill Tunnel, originally constructed in 1884. About 0.4 mile after exiting the tunnel, the trail runs underneath Redwood Highway/US 101, where a recent extension takes users northward past office parks and shopping centers en route to downtown San Rafael. Parts of this segment are bollard-separated on-road bike lanes.

Alternatively, users can travel south from the trail's southern terminus, crossing Corte Madera Creek along a barrier-protected bikeway on US 101 to make additional trail connections.

CONTACT sonomamarintrain.org/smart_pathway

PARKING

Although there are no designated parking lots for this trail, you can reach it via public transit. Bikes are allowed aboard SMART trains, and there are stations at either end of the trail: the **LARKSPUR STATION** (600 Larkspur Landing Cir.; 37.9476, -122.5127), 0.2 mile north of the trail's southern endpoint, and the **SAN RAFAEL STATION** (680 Third St.; 37.9720, -122.5226), 0.1 mile north of the trail's northern endpoint.

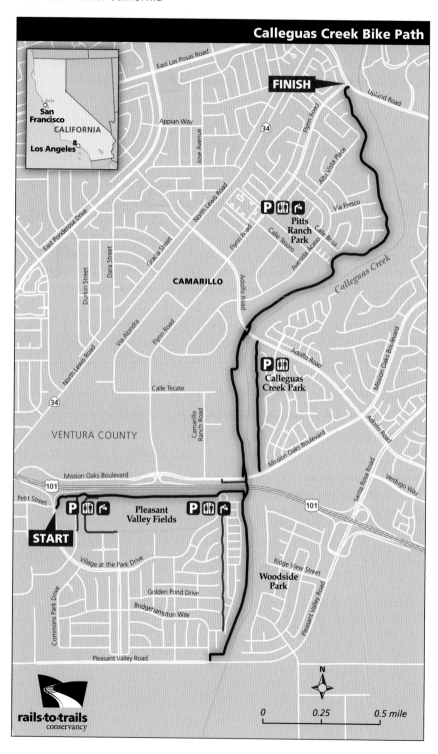

Calleguas Creek Bike Path

Tucked away in aptly named Pleasant Valley at the foot of the Conejo Hills some 50 miles from Los Angeles, the small town of Camarillo boasts 300 days of sunshine annually and many opportunities for fun, such as visiting the Calleguas (pronounced ky-YAY-gas) Creek Bike Path. This 4.4-mile trail traces Calleguas Creek in the eastern part of Camarillo and provides views of the surrounding foothills as well as the namesake creek, an ephemeral stream that runs only when fed sufficient rainwater. The creek is part of the 343-square-mile Calleguas Creek Watershed in Ventura County and is home to a variety of plant and animal life, including low-lying greenery, the occasional shady tree, and 370 bird species. Abundant signage provides information about the area's bird biodiversity along with route guidance.

The paved bike path can also host walkers, runners, and in-line skaters along its undulating route. Note that some of its hills could be challenging for wheelchairs. The

County
Ventura

Endpoints
Village at the Park Dr. and Petit St. (Camarillo); Pleasant Valley Road and Bridgehampton Way (Camarillo); Upland Road and Flynn Road (Camarillo); Adolfo Road, 500 feet west of Rancho Calleguas Dr. (Camarillo); Mission Oaks Blvd., 0.1 mile west of Rancho Calleguas Dr. (Camarillo)

Mileage
4.4

Type
Greenway/Non-Rail-Trail

Roughness Rating
1

Surface
Asphalt

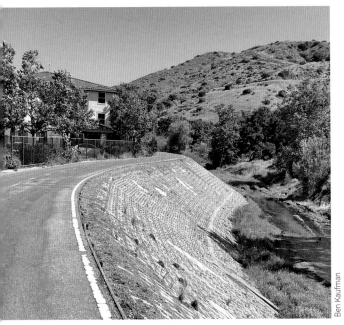

Ben Kaufman

The route traces Calleguas Creek, part of the 343-square-mile Calleguas Creek Watershed.

path is managed by the city and enables visitors and residents to conveniently explore local neighborhoods, schools, and parks.

Our route starts at the Pleasant Valley Fields, where ample parking (more than 600 spots), restrooms, and drinking water are available. Located near a school and family YMCA, the 55-acre park is equipped with playground equipment, picnic areas, lighted sports fields, a snack bar during events, and a paved pathway to allow for easy navigation around the fields.

The trail runs for 0.9 mile from west to east on the north side of the park to the Kingdom Hall of Jehovah's Witnesses, where it arrives at a T junction at Calleguas Creek for the 2.6-mile north–south trail segment.

Those turning south can take the trail for approximately 1 mile along the creek's west bank to its endpoint at Pleasant Valley Road and Bridgehampton Way. About halfway down, Woodside Park can be seen to the east.

Heading north from the T junction, users will pass beneath US 101 and then between the creekbed and the back of a business district. About 1.1 mile north of US 101, a side trail on the left connects to Cedarbrook Walk, which ends in 0.1 mile at Pitts Ranch Park. Another of the town's 28 parks, this 10-acre landscaped facility has restrooms, drinking fountains, and parking. Returning to the trail, visitors will trace a residential area for another mile north to the end at Upland Road.

An unattached, 0.5-mile trail segment that runs along the east side of Calleguas Creek can be reached via the bridges at Adolfo Road or Mission Oaks Boulevard. The 3-acre Calleguas Creek Park is located at the northern end of this section and has a drinking fountain, a playground, and picnic tables.

CONTACT rtc.li/calleguas-creek-bike-path

PARKING

Parking areas are located within Camarillo and are listed from southwest to northeast.
Indicates that at least one accessible parking space is available.

PLEASANT VALLEY FIELDS* Westpark Ct., 0.2 mile north of Village at the Park Dr. (34.2142, -119.0280).

PLEASANT VALLEY FIELDS* Village at the Park Dr., 200 feet west of Calle De La Rosa (34.2152, -119.0180).

PITTS RANCH PARK* 1400 Flynn Road (34.2315, -119.0113).

Community support was integral to the creation of the Sugar Pine and Clovis Old Town Trails, two adjoining rail-trails that link the northern edge of Fresno to southern Clovis. Joggers, cyclists, businesses, and environmental organizations came together to support the development of the trails, which connect many existing area resources, including shops, restaurants, and parks. Through tree-planting efforts organized by the Coalition for Community Trails, about 4,400 trees offer shade and beautiful scenery.

The 4-mile Sugar Pine Trail begins on East Nees Avenue under Yosemite Freeway/CA 41, near the River Park Shopping Center, a large mall complex. The trailhead is under the overpass and is equipped with benches and a drinking fountain. There is ample parking and a wide selection of eateries at the mall across the street. Heading northeast, the trail parallels Cole Avenue and then

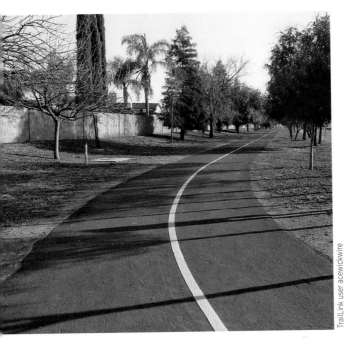

The trail provides access to residential and commercial areas, as well as Clovis's historic downtown.

TrailLink user acewickwire

County
Fresno

Endpoints
E. Nees Ave. under
Yosemite Freeway/
CA 41 (Fresno); E. Copper
Ave. and N. Willow Ave.
(Fresno); Clovis Ave.,
0.2 mile north of
E. Shields Ave. (Clovis)

Mileage
9.6

Type
Rail-Trail

Roughness Rating
1

Surface
Asphalt

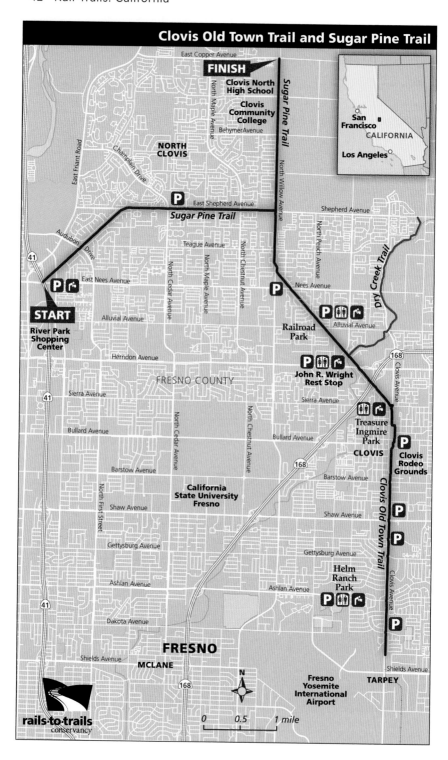

Clovis Old Town Trail and Sugar Pine Trail

continues east on Shepherd Avenue through residential parts of northern Fresno on a wide and spacious corridor bordered by mature trees. Underpasses carry the trail through busy intersections. Additional restaurants and stores are within walking distance of the trail along Shepherd Avenue. At North Willow Avenue, the trail turns south, meeting the Clovis Old Town Trail between East Teague and West Nees Avenues. A segment of the Sugar Pine Trail also travels north along Willow Avenue, passing Clovis Community College and Clovis North High School before ending at East Copper Avenue.

The 5.6-mile Clovis Old Town Trail skirts many residential and commercial areas, with easy access, several parks, and rest-stop shelters with various amenities along its entire length. In the city of Clovis itself, users are afforded convenient access to the community's historical downtown, as well as the Clovis Rodeo Grounds, home to an April rodeo held annually since 1914.

Take the Clovis Old Town Trail southeast into Clovis. Roughly 0.9 mile south of the trail's northern endpoint is Railroad Park, on the corner of Peach

The Coalition for Community Trails has added about 4,400 trees to the route. TrailLink user tucker.furguy

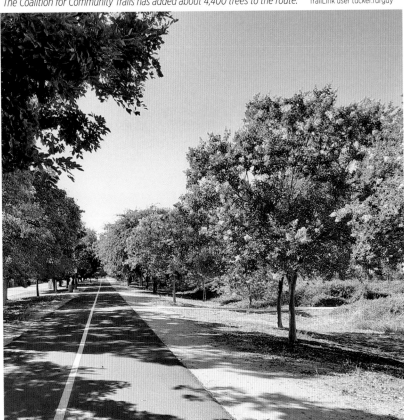

and Alluvial Avenues. This neighborhood park has picnic pavilions, restrooms, drinking fountains, and paved trails. In another 0.6 mile, just after North Villa Avenue, is the John R. Wright Rest Stop, behind the City of Clovis Fire Station 3. Here, you'll find picnic pavilions, restrooms, drinking fountains, and a map display board.

Just south of the rest stop is a connection to the 2.5-mile Dry Creek Trail, which heads northeast to connect to the 2.4-mile Enterprise Canal Trail. Roughly 0.9 mile south of the Dry Creek Trail connection is Treasure Ingmire Park, another community park where you can find picnic pavilions, restrooms, and drinking fountains. About 2.7 miles south of Treasure Ingmire Park, you'll reach Ashlan Avenue. If you need a break (even though you're close to the end), head a half mile west on Ashlan Avenue to Helm Ranch Park, where you can find picnic pavilions, restrooms, drinking fountains, and wildlife-viewing. Back on the trail, it's only 0.7 mile to the southernmost endpoint.

CONTACT **cityofclovis.com/public-utilities/parks** (Clovis Old Town Trail) and **fresno.gov** (Sugar Pine Trail)

PARKING

Parking areas are listed from northwest to southeast. *Indicates that at least one accessible parking space is available.*

FRESNO* River Park Shopping Center, 71 E. Via la Plata (36.8513, -119.7876); park as close to E. Nees Ave. as possible.

FRESNO* E. Champlain Dr. and E. Shepherd Ave. (36.8672, -119.7563).

CLOVIS* Parkway Trails Shopping Center, 1205–1365 N. Willow Ave. (36.8526, -119.7271); trail access is at the northeast corner of N. Willow and W. Nees Aves.

CLOVIS* John R. Wright Rest Stop, small parking lot (6 spaces) behind the City of Clovis Fire Station 3, on N. Minnewawa Ave. between Birch Ave. and Park Creek Dr. (36.8400, -119.7111).

CLOVIS* Clovis Old Town Trail, between Fifth St. and Rodeo Dr. (36.8227, -119.6996).

CLOVIS* Clovis and Shaw Aves. (36.8093, -119.6998); commercial lot with trail access.

CLOVIS* Clovis and Santa Ana Aves. (36.8069, -119.6998); mall parking lot with trail access.

CLOVIS* Helm Ranch Park, Ashlan and Minnewawa Aves. (36.7943, -119.7107).

CLOVIS* Clovis Recreation Center, 3495 Clovis Ave. (36.7885, -119.6998).

Located in the East Bay region of the San Francisco Bay Area, the Contra Costa Canal Regional Trail follows the Contra Costa Canal in a horseshoe shape from Martinez south through Pleasant Hill and Walnut Creek and then east and north to Concord. The canal is a 47-mile aqueduct that was built between 1937 and 1948. It's used as a residential, agricultural, and industrial water supply for almost a dozen communities along the canal. Because it's part of the water supply system, the canal is fenced off, with no access for fishing or other water-based recreation. The canal is a vital part of the community infrastructure, and the trail built alongside it allows myriad access points to the surrounding neighborhoods and business districts.

The paved pathway winds through a diverse array of settings, including neighborhoods, school campuses, parks, and light industrial areas. Much of the trail is tree lined, with several scenic vistas of mountain peaks and

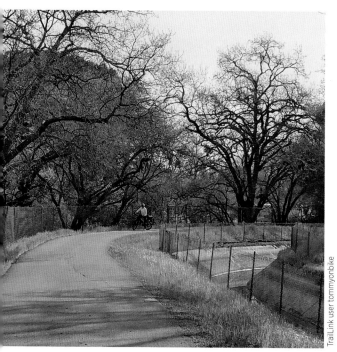

TrailLink user tommyonbike

The trail traces an early 20th-century canal in a horseshoe shape from Martinez to Concord.

County
Contra Costa

Endpoints
Muir Road, 0.2 mile west of Pacheco Blvd. (Martinez); Willow Pass Road, 340 feet east of Sixth St. (Concord)

Mileage
13.8

Type
Greenway/Non-Rail-Trail

Roughness Rating
1

Surface
Asphalt, Concrete

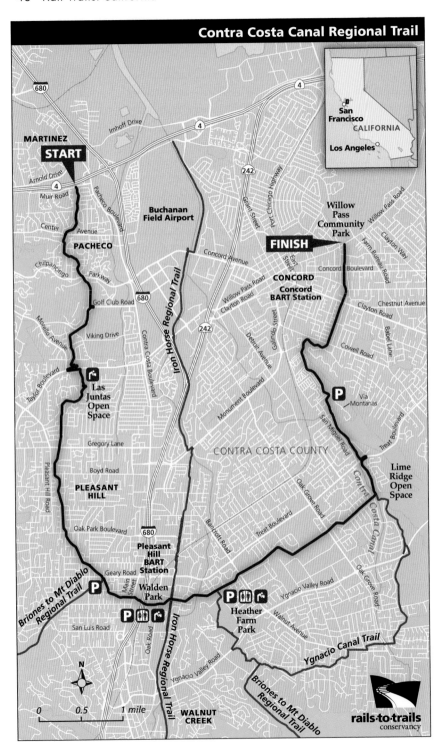

Contra Costa Canal Regional Trail

San Francisco
CALIFORNIA
Los Angeles

680

Imhoff Drive

4

4

MARTINEZ
START

242

Arnold Drive

4

Muir Road

Pacheco Boulevard

Buchanan Field Airport

Concord Avenue

Willow Pass Road

Port Chicago Highway

Willow Pass Community Park

Willow Pass Road

Clayton Way

Center

Avenue

PACHECO

FINISH

East Street

Farm Bureau Road

Chilpancingo

Parkway

Iron Horse Regional Trail

Grant Street

CONCORD
Concord BART Station

Concord Boulevard

Chestnut Avenue

Clayton Road

680

Golf Club Road

Willow Pass Road

Clayton Road

Galindo Street

Babel Lane

Morello Avenue

Viking Drive

Contra Costa Boulevard

242

Detroit Avenue

Cowell Road

Las Juntas Open Space

P

Via Montanas

Treat Boulevard

Taylor Boulevard

Gregory Lane

CONTRA COSTA COUNTY

San Miguel Road

Lime Ridge Open Space

Boyd Road

PLEASANT HILL

Contra Costa Canal

Pleasant Hill Road

Oak Park Boulevard

680

Bancroft Road

Treat Boulevard

Oak Grove Road

Oak Grove Road

Pleasant Hill BART Station

Briones to Mt Diablo Regional Trail

P

Geary Road

Walden Park

Ygnacio Valley Road

Main Street

P

P

Heather Farm Park

Walnut Avenue

San Luis Road

Oak Road

Iron Horse Regional Trail

Ygnacio Valley Road

Ygnacio Canal Trail

Oak Grove Road

N

Briones to Mt Diablo Regional Trail

0   0.5   1 mile

WALNUT CREEK

rails·to·trails
conservancy

rolling hills. The canal itself attracts a variety of wildlife, including many bird species. There are multiple road crossings, but they are all well-marked, and the more heavily trafficked intersections have crosswalk buttons.

With several parks dotting the route, it's relatively easy to find a restroom or a place to refill a water bottle. Beginning from the trail's west end, you'll encounter your first one, Las Juntas Open Space, in 3.2 miles. In another 3.6 miles, you'll reach Walden Park, near the trail's midpoint, which offers a playground and sports facilities, including a basketball court and a disc golf course. In another 0.9 mile, you'll reach Heather Farm Park, a popular outdoor space with a garden center, a fishing pond, an equestrian center (equestrian use is permitted on the Contra Costa trail as well), and other recreational amenities. Continuing northeast for 2.4 miles, you'll reach the western boundary of Lime Ridge Open Space, a more than 1,200-acre natural oasis with more trails to explore. After your final 3.7 miles, the trail ends at Willow Pass Road with Willow Pass Community Park across the street.

Several trails connect to the Costa Contra Canal Regional Trail, most notably the 32-mile Iron Horse Regional Trail (see page 99), which bisects the canal trail at about its midpoint. The 5.7-mile Ygnacio Canal Trail offers an opportunity for a loop, connecting with the Costa Contra Canal Regional Trail in two places: at Heather Farm Park and again at Lime Ridge Open Space. The Briones to Mt. Diablo Regional Trail (which includes some unpaved sections) joins the Costa Contra Canal Regional Trail at the bottom of the horseshoe and continues west to Briones Regional Park and southeast to Diablo Foothills Regional Park.

CONTACT ebparks.org/trails/interpark/contra-costa-canal

PARKING

Parking areas are listed from west to east. *Indicates that at least one accessible parking space is available.*

WALNUT CREEK* EBMUD Trail Park and Staging on Geary Road, 450 feet east of Buena Vista Ave./Putnam Blvd. (37.9268, -122.0715).

WALNUT CREEK* Walden Park, 2698 Oak Road (37.9214, -122.0580).

WALNUT CREEK* Heather Farm Park, 301 N. San Carlos Dr. (37.9222, -122.0433).

CONCORD Lime Ridge Open Space on Via Montanas, 0.3 mile northeast of San Miguel Road (37.9574, -122.0207).

The trail is also close to two Bay Area Rapid Transit (BART) stations: **PLEASANT HILL/ CONTRA COSTA CENTRE** (1365 Treat Blvd., Walnut Creek; 37.9284, -122.05598), near the trail's midpoint, and **CONCORD** (1451 Oakland Ave., Concord; 37.9737, -122.0293), near its eastern terminus.

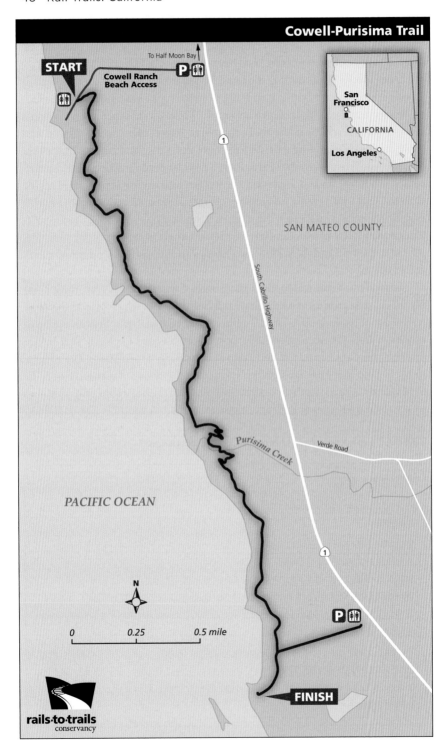

Cowell-Purisima Trail

To Half Moon Bay

START

Cowell Ranch
Beach Access

P

San
Francisco

CALIFORNIA

Los Angeles

SAN MATEO COUNTY

South Cabrillo Highway

Purisima Creek

Verde Road

PACIFIC OCEAN

N

0   0.25   0.5 mile

P

FINISH

rails·to·trails
conservancy

Just south of Half Moon Bay, the Cowell-Purisima Trail would be a worthy addition to any avid trail user's bucket list. As part of the California Coastal Trail—a network of bicycling and hiking trails that, when complete, will stretch along the coastline for 1,230 miles from Oregon to the Mexican border—this 4.1-mile pathway is possibly one of the most beautiful trails in the state. Originating as private family farmland and developed in 2010, it features stunning, unobstructed views of the Pacific Ocean for most of your journey.

The Cowell-Purisima Trail is rich with history. The land that the trail was created on has been a working farm since the mid-1800s. In 1988, the Peninsula Open Space Trust (POST) acquired the Cowell family ranch with a mission to protect the coastline and allow farming to continue by selling most of the land to local farmers. The trail is now managed by San Mateo County Parks.

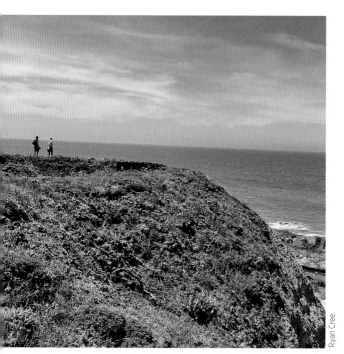

With sweeping Pacific views, the trail offers a quintessential California experience.

Ryan Cree

County
San Mateo

Endpoints
Cabrillo Hwy./CA 1, just south of Dehoff Canyon Road (Half Moon Bay); Cabrillo Hwy./CA 1, 0.6 mile south of Verde Road (Half Moon Bay)

Mileage
4.1

Type
Greenway/Non-Rail-Trail

Roughness Rating
1–2

Surface
Dirt, Gravel

You should probably plan on parking at the northern section of the trail, which maintains a more consistent schedule of opening daily from 8 a.m. to 5 p.m., although the farmers who own the land reserve the right to close the trail at any time for specific purposes related to their farm work, such as moving animals or watering fields.

Although most of the trail is accessible, a small middle section contains steep terrain that would make it extremely difficult for any nonmotorized-wheelchair user to make it through without assistance. It is recommended that wheelchair users park at either end of the trail (north or south) and return to their start point once they reach the challenging terrain.

On your trek from the northern parking lot to quite nearly the water's edge at the southern end, you will travel along a small private farm road and, depending on the time of year, may notice a vast valley of budding Brussels sprouts. As you travel south along the gravel trail, you'll find yourself sandwiched between the Pacific Ocean and the Cowell Ranch Farm, as well as other historical

As you travel the trail, you'll be sandwiched between the ocean and historical farmland.   Joe LaCroix

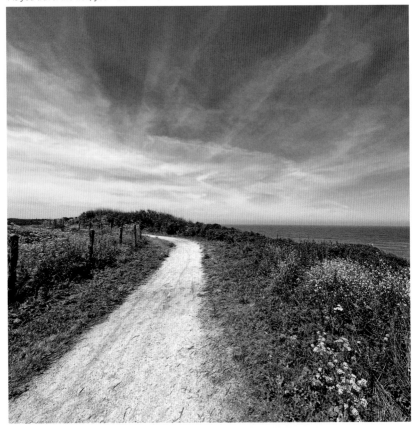

family-owned farms. Here, the trail is immersed in an agricultural setting with picturesque farmland and domestic animals dotting the landscape. As the trail begins to parallel the Pacific coastline, enjoy the vistas of elevated rocky cliffs visible for miles.

The most difficult section of the trail lies between mile 1.75 and mile 2, where the grade is steep and the hillside route is so winding that an average bike rider would need to dismount to proceed. Luckily, this section is short enough that it doesn't present a major concern. Over the next mile, you'll follow the coastline again with breathtaking views of the protected beaches that are home to local harbor seals. The last 0.6 mile continues to wind through vegetable fields and cow pastures and along the Pacific until you reach the southern trailhead. The trail extends just a little beyond a turnoff for a parking area and features another sightseeing spot with expansive views of the water and cliffs.

CONTACT smcgov.org/parks/cowell-purisima-trail

PARKING

Parking areas are located within Half Moon Bay and are listed from north to south. *Indicates that at least one accessible parking space is available.*

COWELL RANCH BEACH ACCESS PARKING* Cabrillo Hwy./CA 1, just south of Dehoff Canyon Road (37.4221, -122.4264).

COWELL-PURISIMA TRAIL PARKING* Cabrillo Hwy./CA 1, 0.6 mile south of Verde Road (37.3963, -122.4157).

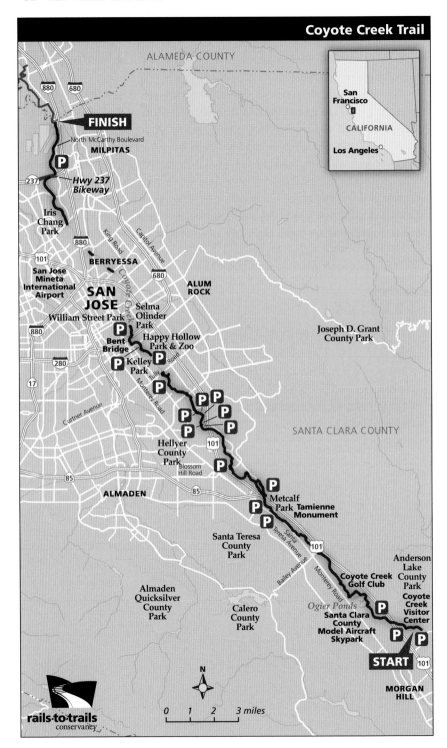

Coyote Creek Trail

A TRAIL NATION PROJECT

Stretching from Morgan Hill up to the southern extent of the San Francisco Bay, the Coyote Creek Trail is one of the longest trails in San Jose. More than 25 miles are currently open in three main segments and several smaller segments. When complete, it will span more than 30 miles, following Coyote Creek for most of the way. The trail is part of a developing 2,600-miles-plus Bay Area regional trail network being spearheaded by the Bay Area Trails Collaborative (**railstotrails.org/bay-area**) and Rails-to-Trails Conservancy as a TrailNation™ project to increase safe walking, biking, and trail access for millions of Bay Area residents.

As of spring 2023, the completed segments of the Coyote Creek Trail are as follows:

➤ Eagle View Dr. and Morning Star Dr. (Morgan Hill) to Tully Community Ballfields, Tully Road and Galveston Ave. (San Jose)

➤ Basking Ridge Ave., 0.1 mile south of Veranda Way (San Jose) to Basking Ridge Ave. and Silicon Valley Blvd.

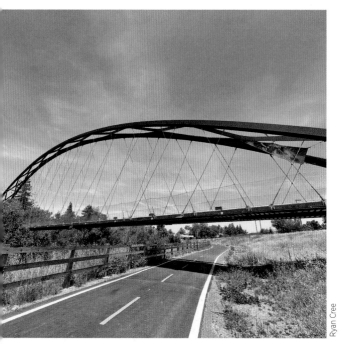

Ryan Cree

Spanning 25-plus miles, the Coyote Creek Trail is one of the longest trails in San José.

County
Santa Clara

Endpoints
Eagle View Dr. and Morning Star Dr. (Morgan Hill); N. McCarthy Blvd., 0.3 mile south of Dixon Landing Road (Milpitas)
Full list of endpoints in the description

Mileage
25.6

Type
Greenway/Non-Rail-Trail

Roughness Rating
1

Surface
Asphalt, Crushed Stone

➤ Kelley Park, Phelan Ave. and Roberts Ave. (San Jose) to Selma Olinder Park at E. William St. between Brookwood Ave. and S. 18th St. (San Jose)

➤ Mercado Way and Berryessa Road (San Jose) to just past Mercado Way, near Chessington Dr. (San Jose)

➤ Old Oakland Road between Schallenberger Road and Pear Orchard Dr. (San Jose) to Pear Orchard Dr. and Elderflower Pl. (San Jose)

➤ Montague Expressway, near Kruse Dr. (San Jose) to CA 237/Southbay Fwy., 0.6 mile east of Zanker Road (Milpitas)

➤ Alviso Milpitas Road and Ranch Dr. (Milpitas) to N. McCarthy Blvd., 0.3 mile south of Dixon Landing Road (Milpitas)

Begin your journey at the southern endpoint of the trail, which starts at the intersection of Morning Star and Eagle View Drives, a couple hundred feet from the Coyote Creek Visitor Center at Anderson Lake County Park, where parking is available. This longest segment of completed trail—at approximately 18.7 miles—heads north and soon parallels its namesake waterway. There is a parallel foot/equestrian trail for the next half mile until Burnett Avenue, where riders will find a staging area and the beginning of an equestrian trail. (For a map of this trail, including water troughs and other staging areas, please see **rtc.li /coyote-trail-map.**)

Watch out for hobbyists flying model airplanes as you pass the Santa Clara County Model Aircraft Skypark. At Ogier Ponds, you can spy a rich diversity of birdlife and perhaps even catch a few *birdies* as the trail passes the Coyote Creek Golf Club. Following the club is the Tamienne Monument, a trailside plaque inscribed in binary code that marks the center of the Santa Clara Valley. Immediately following the monument, south of Metcalf Road, the equestrian trail comes to an end. You'll pass Metcalf Park, after which the trail becomes more urban as it enters the southern reaches of the city of San Jose, though it remains largely riparian. After Hellyer County Park, continue another 2.5 miles to Tully Road.

To reach the second, 2-mile trail segment, turn right onto Tully Road and then left onto Lucretia Avenue, with its well-marked bike lanes. In 0.8 mile, turn left onto Phelan Avenue and pick the trail up again in about 0.1 mile at Roberts Avenue. This portion of trail, which opened in 2021, traverses Kelley Park, where it connects to the nearby Happy Hollow Park & Zoo during park hours by way of the arcing Bent Bridge. Cross Story Road to continue along the trail, passing under a historical railway trestle (closed to the public) and through Selma Olinder and William Street Parks to where this segment ends at East William Street.

The northernmost, 4.9-mile section technically begins at Montague Expressway but is not directly accessible for another 0.4 mile north, at Iris Chang Park.

The trail continues along a crushed-stone pathway atop a levee above the south-western bank of Coyote Creek next to a residential area. The trail soon changes back to asphalt and meets the Highway 237 Bikeway at the Southbay Freeway/ CA 237. Merge right onto the trail and turn left to cross at McCarthy Boulevard, where the trail picks up again to the left, off Ranch Drive. The pathway continues north through an industrial area to North McCarthy Boulevard.

CONTACT sanjose.org/listings/coyote-creek-trail

PARKING

Parking areas are listed from south to north. Select parking areas for the trail are listed below. For a detailed list of parking areas and other waypoints, go to **TrailLink.com™**. *Indicates that at least one accessible parking space is available.*

MORGAN HILL* Coyote Creek Visitor Center at Anderson Lake County Park, 19245 Malaguerra Ave. (37.1669, -121.6496).

SAN JOSE* Metcalf Park, Monterey Hwy. and Forsum Road (37.2295, -121.7574).

SAN JOSE* Silver Creek Valley Road near Piercy Road (37.2575, -121.7911).

SAN JOSE* Hellyer County Park, Palisade Dr. and Hellyer Ave. (37.2833, -121.8128); day-use fees may apply.

SAN JOSE* Tully Road, between Galveston Ave. and La Ragione Ave. (37.3105, -121.8429).

SAN JOSE* Selma Olinder Park, E. William St., between Brookwood Ave. and S. 18th St. (37.3375, -121.8677).

SAN JOSE Iris Chang Park, Epic Way, 0.4 mile north of Montague Expy. (37.4005, -121.9193); limited on-street parking.

MILPITAS Ranch Dr. and McCarthy Blvd. (37.4258, -121.9249).

MILPITAS* 1425 N. McCarthy Blvd. (37.4471, -121.9225).

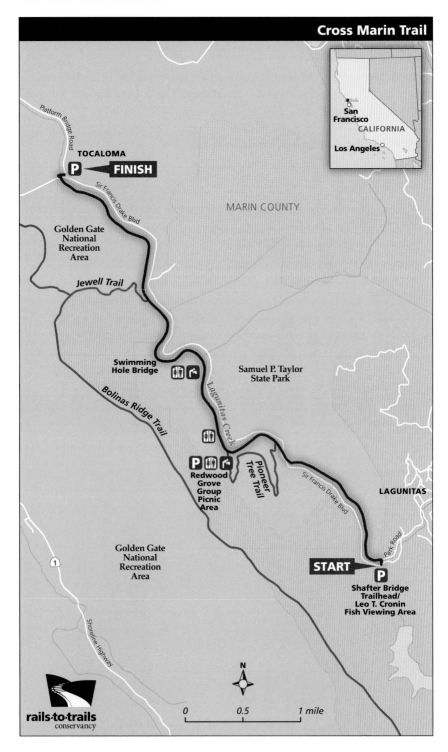

Cross Marin Trail

CALIFORNIA

San Francisco

Los Angeles

Platform Bridge Road

TOCALOMA

P ◄ FINISH

Sir Francis Drake Blvd

MARIN COUNTY

Golden Gate
National
Recreation
Area

Jewell Trail

Swimming
Hole Bridge

Bolinas Ridge Trail

Lagunitas Creek

Samuel P. Taylor
State Park

Redwood
Grove
Group
Picnic
Area

Pioneer
Tree Trail

Sir Francis Drake Blvd

LAGUNITAS

Park Road

Golden Gate
National
Recreation
Area

START P

Shafter Bridge
Trailhead/
Leo T. Cronin
Fish Viewing Area

Shoreline Highway

1

N

rails·to·trails
conservancy

0   0.5   1 mile

The spectacular Cross Marin Trail, also known as the Sir Francis Drake Bikeway, follows the route of the former North Pacific Coast Railroad and roughly parallels the sinuous Sir Francis Drake Boulevard. The family-friendly, partly paved rail-trail makes up a segment of Northern California's Bay Area Ridge Trail, which in turn is part of a developing 2,600-miles-plus Bay Area regional trail network being spearheaded by the Bay Area Trails Collaborative (**railsto trails.org/bay-area**) and Rails-to-Trails Conservancy as a TrailNation™ project to increase safe walking, biking, and trail access for millions of Bay Area residents.

On its southern end, the trail begins as a gravel-and-dirt path in the dense woodlands of Lagunitas. While small footbridges ensure users have a safe path over culvert overflows, this unpaved section of trail is not suitable for wheelchair use. On your left are thick redwood stands cushioned by sorrel and ferns, as is the lovely Lagunitas

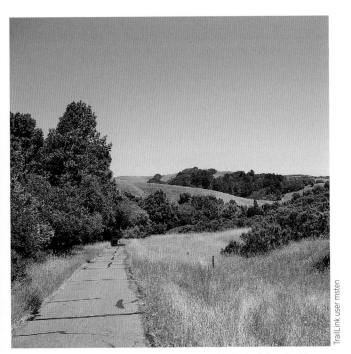

A state park and other recreational areas provide the backdrop for this scenic pathway.

TrailLink user msten

County
Marin

Endpoints
Sir Francis Drake Blvd., 0.3 mile west of Park Road (Lagunitas); Platform Bridge Road, just north of Sir Francis Drake Blvd. (Tocaloma)

Mileage
5.3

Type
Rail-Trail

Roughness Rating
1–2

Surface
Asphalt, Dirt, Gravel

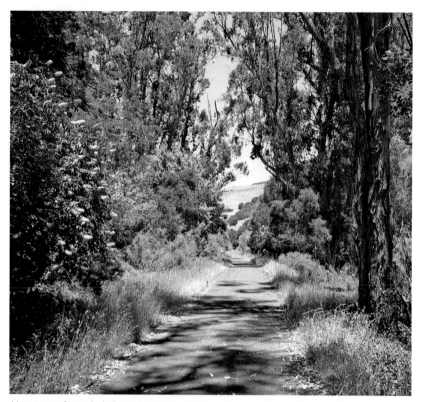

Many types of trees, including oak, madrone, laurel, and Douglas-fir, are visible along the trail.
TrailLink user msten

Creek (closed from December to mid-June for salmon protection). At mile 1.5, you arrive at a bridge carrying trail traffic over both Sir Francis Drake Boulevard and Lagunitas Creek. A cheeky red SALMON CROSSING sign alerts trailgoers to threatened populations of silver (or coho) salmon and steelhead trout that migrate up the creek to spawn during the winter. This is the first of several spots along the trail where you can view them (and possibly, beavers that sometimes work in the area).

Just past the bridge is an unmarked and easy to miss intersection with the 1.6-mile Pioneer Tree Trail, a hiking and equestrian path that rejoins our trail at mile 2. Here, you'll go through a gate that leads to the paved and lightly trafficked on-road section of the trail as it goes through Samuel P. Taylor State Park. Samuel Taylor was an entrepreneur who struck it rich during the California gold rush and created Camp Taylor, one of the first sites in the country to offer camping as a recreational activity. In the 1870s and 1880s, it was common for families to take the railroad out to the camp for the weekend.

You'll pass the Redwood Grove Group Picnic Area, followed by several campsites that, while frequently full, do not detract from the area's natural beauty. Oak, tanoak, madrone, live oak, laurel, and Douglas-fir are all visible along the path, which is lined with California native buttercups, Indian paintbrush, and milkmaids. Black-tailed deer, the most common animal in the state park, can often be spotted from the trail.

The final section is shaded by cool redwood groves. For a quick detour and dip in the creek, veer right at mile 3.1 to the popular Swimming Hole Bridge. Another 0.8 mile north of the swimming hole, you'll intersect the Jewell Trail, a 1-mile connector to the 11-mile Bolinas Ridge Trail. From here, the remainder of the Cross Marin Trail is located in the Golden Gate National Recreation Area.

To extend your day, try exploring the numerous other trails in Samuel P. Taylor State Park (day-use fees apply year-round). Horseback riding is allowed on the entirety of the trail. Public equestrian parking is available along Sir Francis Drake Boulevard via large pullouts.

CONTACT rtc.li/samuel-p-taylor-sp

PARKING

Parking areas are listed from south to north. *Indicates that at least one accessible parking space is available.*

LAGUNITAS* Shafter Bridge Trailhead/Leo T. Cronin Fish Viewing Area, Sir Francis Drake Blvd., 0.3 mile west of Park Road (38.0041, -122.7090); small parking lot with a 1-hour limit.

LAGUNITAS* Redwood Grove Group Picnic Area, dead end of Taylor Park Road, 0.3 mile southwest of Samuel P. Taylor State Park entrance (38.0180, -122.7331).

TOCALOMA Old Sir Francis Drake Blvd. and Taylor Park Road, across the road from a historical bridge closed to vehicle traffic (38.0501, -122.7604).

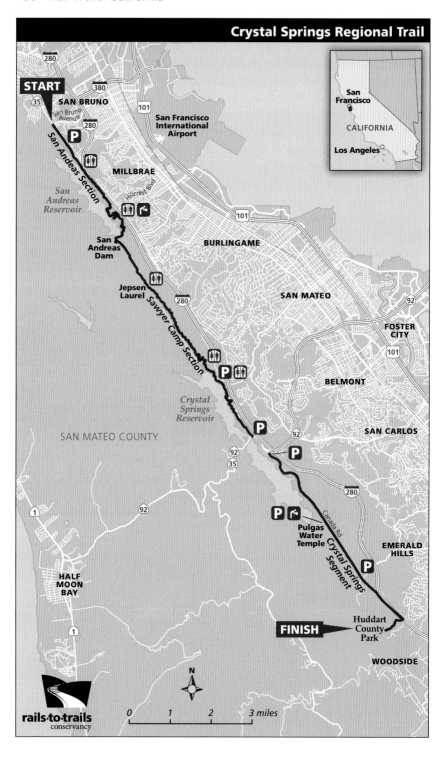

Crystal Springs Regional Trail

The Crystal Springs Regional Trail offers tranquil views of two long, narrow reservoirs and a lake that sit atop the San Andreas Rift Zone, a geologic fault that shook violently in the destructive 1906 San Francisco earthquake and others.

The trail runs down a ridge on the San Francisco Peninsula between San Bruno and Woodside and consists of three sections: (from north to south) the 2.6-mile San Andreas section and the 7.2-mile Sawyer Camp section, which make up a connected segment intersecting near where I-280 exits onto Hillcrest Boulevard in Millbrae, and the 6.7-mile Crystal Springs segment.

The two contiguous northern segments are mostly wide, paved, and reasonably graded, except for the southernmost 0.6-mile section of the San Andreas segment. Due to the steeper grade and narrow gravel surface, this stretch is accessible only to walkers and equestrians. To avoid it, bicyclists, skaters, and wheelchair users are directed to

County
San Mateo

Endpoints
San Andreas/Sawyer Camp segment: San Bruno Ave. W. and Skyline Blvd. (San Bruno); Skyline Blvd. and CA 92/Half Moon Bay Road (San Mateo) *Crystal Springs segment:* CA 92/Half Moon Bay Road and Cañada Road (San Mateo); Huddart County Park at Raymundo Dr., 200 feet north of Marva Oaks Dr. (Woodside)

Mileage
16.5

Type
Greenway/Non-Rail-Trail

Roughness Rating
1–3

Surface
Asphalt, Gravel, Dirt

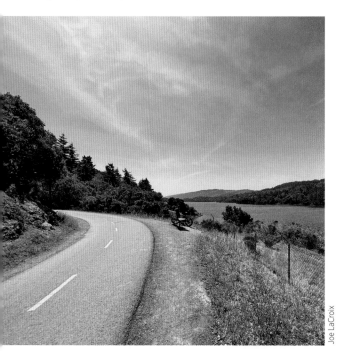

Joe LaCroix

The trail offers expansive views of two narrow reservoirs and a lake.

take Skyline Boulevard via Larkspur Drive and Hillcrest Boulevard. The Crystal Springs segment is dirt and open only to walkers and horse riders. It is maintained by San Mateo County, which does not allow pets.

The northernmost trailhead with parking is located a half mile south of the trail endpoint at San Bruno Avenue. The San Andreas section features views of San Andreas Reservoir at the foot of Sweeney Ridge.

The Sawyer Camp section begins at Hillcrest Boulevard. It's considered the busiest trail section in San Mateo County and has a posted speed limit of 15 miles per hour. Spanish explorers followed this route in the 16th century, and it later became a wagon road that led to a lodge operated in the mid-1800s by landowner Leander Sawyer. The trail heads downhill and away from the interstate at the southern end of the San Andreas Reservoir and crosses a dam. You'll pass through a forest that offers shade and places for picnicking. This area is also home to deer and other wildlife, as well as the Jepson laurel, said to be 600 years old and the largest such tree in the state.

The Crystal Springs Reservoir emerges about 2.3 miles past the dam, offering pleasant views in clearings for the next 4.5 miles to the end of the Sawyer

With its jaw-dropping scenery, Crystal Springs Regional Trail is one of the most popular routes in San Mateo County.   Joe LaCroix

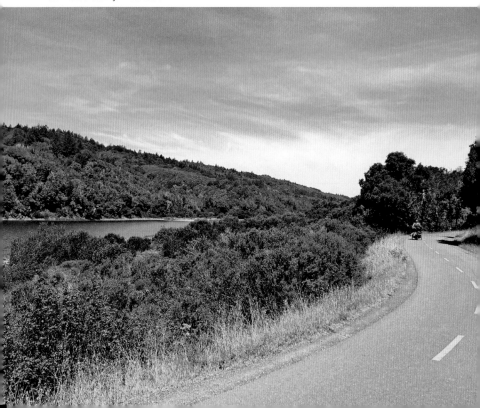

Camp section at CA 35/Skyline Boulevard and CA 92/Half Moon Bay Road. A dam here separates the upper and lower reservoirs.

The Crystal Springs segment begins 0.5 mile south on CA 92 at Cañada Road. This dirt track on the western side of the right-of-way is suitable only for hiking, jogging, and equestrian use. Bicyclists can use the shoulder of Cañada Road in this area.

In 2.3 miles, the Pulgas Water Temple serves as an intriguing destination consisting of a Corinthian-columned temple erected by the City of San Francisco to commemorate the achievement of bringing water to the area. Visitors can refill their water bottles straight from the spring. In 2.5 miles, the trail runs alongside I-280 and then turns southwest for a mile to the boundary of 974-acre Huddart Park.

Closure Notice: Due to the 2022–2023 storms, the Sawyer Camp and San Andreas segments of the Crystal Springs Regional Trail are closed due to fallen trees and other storm damage. Visit **rtc.li/san-mateo** for details.

CONTACT smcgov.org/parks/crystal-springs-regional-trail

PARKING

Parking areas are listed from north to south. Select parking areas for the trail are listed below. For a detailed list of parking areas and other waypoints, go to **TrailLink.com™**. *Indicates that at least one accessible parking space is available.*

SAN BRUNO* CA 35/Skyline Blvd., 0.5 mile southeast of San Bruno Ave. W. (37.6121, -122.4361).

BURLINGAME* Sawyer Camp Trail South Trailhead, CA 35/Skyline Blvd. and Crystal Springs Road (37.5310, -122.3639); lot and roadside.

REDWOOD CITY CA 35/Skyline Blvd. and CA 92/Half Moon Bay Road (37.5122, -122.3499).

REDWOOD CITY Cañada Road, just southwest of CA 92/Half Moon Bay Road (37.5061, -122.3408); roadside parking.

REDWOOD CITY* Pulgas Water Temple, 88 Cañada Road (37.4828, -122.3154); roadside parking.

REDWOOD CITY* Edgewood Road and Cañada Road (37.4640, -122.2974).

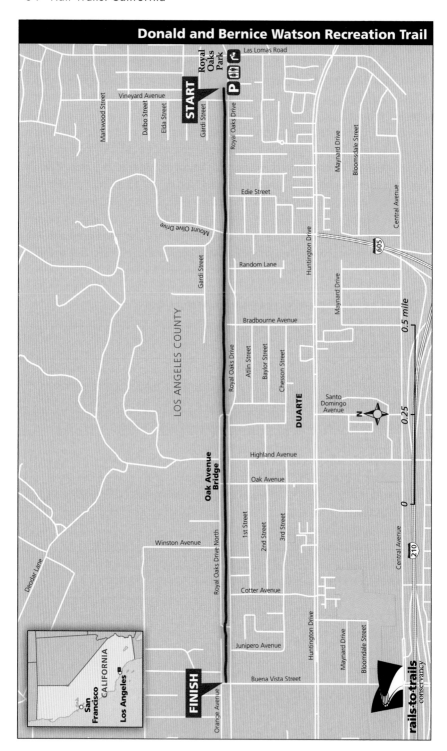

Donald and Bernice Watson Recreation Trail

Nestled on the north side of the sprawling Los Angeles metropolis, the Donald and Bernice Watson Recreation Trail (formerly the Duarte Recreational Trail) runs on parallel asphalt and dirt paths for 1.6 miles through the town of Duarte. Connecting a park, a K–8 school, a medical center, and churches, the trail knits together the community at the foot of the looming San Gabriel Mountains and Angeles National Forest.

The trail follows a short segment of a former electrified trolley system that served the booming Los Angeles, Orange, San Bernardino, and Riverside Counties in the first half of the 20th century. Known locally as the Red Cars, the privately owned Pacific Electric Railway got its start in 1901. It laid more than 1,000 miles of track throughout Southern California, growing with the promise of supplying electricity to far-flung communities.

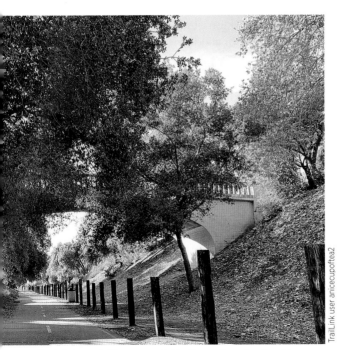

TrailLink user anicecupoftea2

The Oak Avenue bridge once carried traffic over the railroad corridor now serving as a rail-trail.

County
Los Angeles

Endpoints
Royal Oaks Park (Duarte); Buena Vista St., between Orange Ave. and Royal Oaks Dr. (Duarte)

Mileage
1.6

Type
Rail-Trail

Roughness Rating
1

Surface
Asphalt, Dirt

The system declined after World War II with the increased use of automobiles and trucks and the construction of freeways. The system was sold in 1960. Some of the old corridors became rapid transit lines, while housing sprouted on others. This segment through Duarte opened as a trail in 1977 due to the efforts of former Duarte mayor Donald Watson, the first Black city councilman and mayor in the Los Angeles area, and his wife, Bernice.

The city is named for Andres Duarte, a Mexican soldier who was granted 7,000 acres here in 1841 while the area was still under Mexican rule. When the United States gained control of California after the Mexican-American War, Duarte launched a legal battle to retain title to his land grant. The US Supreme Court eventually ruled in his favor in 1878, but by then he had sold his entire ranch piece by piece to pay off debts and legal fees.

The 5-acre Royal Oaks Park, with parking and restrooms, serves as a good starting point at the east end of the trail. You'll notice there's plenty of room on the corridor for both the paved and dirt paths, separated by a series of fence posts. Bicyclists prefer the paved trail, while horseback riders tend to use the dirt trail. Walkers and joggers frequent both. The trail is open from dawn to dusk.

On sunny days, native oaks provide welcome shade. The Indigenous peoples who first settled here 2,500 years ago used acorns from oaks like these to create a flour paste that provided a major part of their diet.

An especially picturesque sight emerges 1.1 mile down the trail as it passes beneath the old arched Oak Avenue Bridge, which once carried traffic over the tracks between Royal Oaks Drive North and Royal Oaks Drive. The bridge is closed to traffic today.

CONTACT accessduarte.com/government/departments/parks-and-recreation

PARKING

Parking is located within Duarte at the east end of the trail. *Indicates that at least one accessible parking space is available.*

ROYAL OAKS PARK* 2627 Royal Oaks Dr. (34.1435, -117.9488).

The Peggy Mensinger Trail is a flat, paved, family-friendly greenway that runs west to east. With neighborhoods to the north and south, it provides a popular gateway for residents. The trail parallels Dry Creek—aptly named, as the rainfall-dependent water flow typically runs quite low. The pathway is narrow, but as the trail meanders from side to side, you never feel restricted. Wildflowers are abundant throughout, and the birdlife is prolific, including yellow-billed magpies, American goldfinches, and Western scrub jays.

If you are planning to drive, the best place to begin is the trail's western endpoint at Moose Park, as the eastern endpoint does not have a parking area. Heading east from the western end, you'll pass through a thick forest of eucalyptus trees running through Kewin Park that offers plentiful shade.

There is a second entrance to the trail north of Dry Creek at the intersection of Scenic Drive and Coffee Road, which also features a parking area with an accessible parking spot. The midway point of the trail, East La Loma Park, offers restrooms, a new playground, tennis courts, a parking area, and a 27-hole disc golf course. The landscape

County
Stanislaus

Endpoints
Moose Park at N. Morton Blvd. and Rue De Yoe (Modesto); south of Scenic Dr., between Coffee Road and Sunnyside Ave. (Modesto); Claus Road and Creekwood Dr. (Modesto)

Mileage
4.7

Type
Greenway/Non-Rail-Trail

Roughness Rating
1

Surface
Asphalt

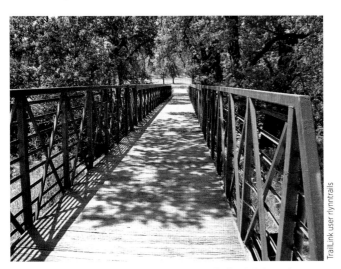

TrailLink user rlynntrails

A pedestrian bridge welcomes trail users near the Scenic Drive and Coffee Road entrance.

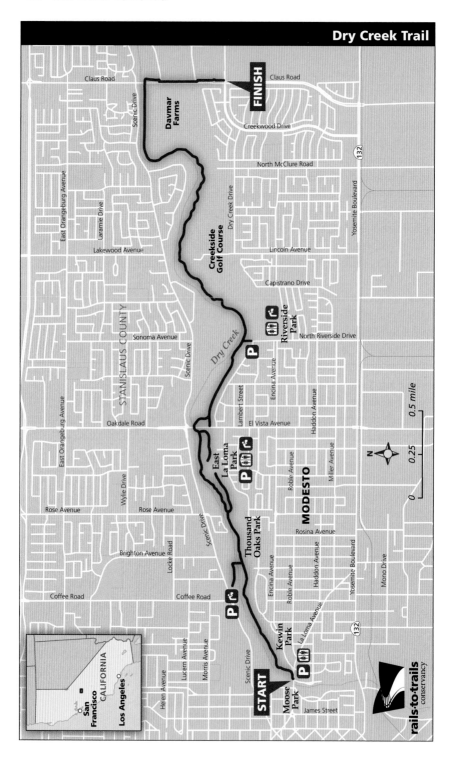

Dry Creek Trail

starts opening up a bit, making it perfect for unimpeded disc golf. Bring plenty of water, especially in the summertime. Leaving the park as you cross under El Vista Avenue, the landscape changes quite dramatically to sandy soil and low bushes, highlighting the semiarid climate of the area.

Traveling farther east will bring you past the expansive public Creekside Golf Course. Once past here, the landscape changes again to a native oak forest to the north and farmland to the south. When you reach the underpass of Claus Road, you'll turn south to reach the eastern endpoint of the trail.

CONTACT rtc.li/modesto-trails

PARKING

Parking areas are located within Modesto and are listed from west to east. *Indicates that at least one accessible parking space is available.*

MOOSE PARK N. Morton Blvd. and Rue De Yoe (37.6444, -120.9846); street parking.

SCENIC DRIVE* Scenic Dr., between Coffee Road and Sunnyside Ave., (37.6489, -120.9751); north of Thousand Oaks Park.

EAST LA LOMA PARK 2001 Edgebrook Dr. (37.6511, -120.9615).

N. RIVERSIDE DRIVE N. Riverside Dr. and Edgebrook Dr. (37.6475, -120.9482); street parking.

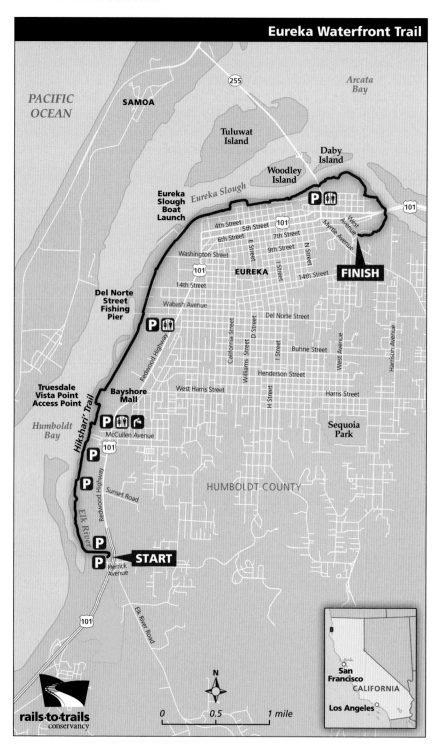

The Eureka Waterfront Trail traces the shorelines of the Elk River and Humboldt Bay for 6.5 miles in this Northern California town. The wide, paved trail, with access to public fishing and water activities, makes it popular with residents and visitors alike. Dotted along the trail are seven benches designed by local artists for the 2018 trail opening. While on the trail, take a moment to learn about the region's history and the people, flora, fauna, and marine life that have called it home.

The southern endpoint is easily accessible via the Herrick Avenue Park & Ride, with views of Elk River and a salt marsh. Time your visit on this portion of the trail by the tide. During high tide you will enjoy a peaceful lagoon, and at low tide you may observe textured mudflats peppered with salt marsh. Avid bird-watchers may spot birds of prey, such as bald eagles and peregrine falcons, as well as songbirds, including the yellow warbler.

Coinciding with the Eureka Waterfront Trail's southern section, the 1.5-mile Hikshari' Trail runs north from

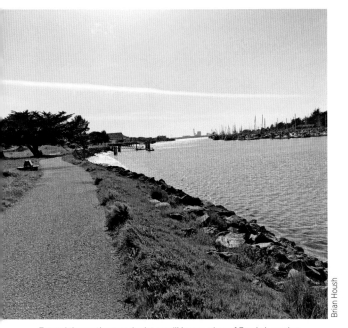

Brian Housh

Toward the northern endpoint, you'll have a view of Eureka's marina.

County
Humboldt

Endpoints
Herrick Ave. Park & Ride at Pound Road and Herrick Ave. (Eureka); Tydd St., several hundred feet northeast of West Ave. (Eureka)

Mileage
6.5

Type
Rail-Trail; Greenway/ Non-Rail-Trail; Rail-with-Trail

Roughness Rating
1

Surface
Asphalt, Boardwalk

the Elk River Wildlife Area, honoring the ancestral homeland of the Wiyot people, who resided in the area for thousands of years. The Hikshari' Trail ends at a trailhead at Truesdale Street, where you'll find a picnic area and other amenities.

As you continue north, the trail follows a former railroad that was a major transportation vein for Eureka's lumber industry. When California's gold rush brought a demand for lumber, the region's natural resource—redwood—was in high demand. By 1854, nine lumber mills operated around Humboldt Bay, making Eureka the largest producer of lumber in the Pacific region. Signs of the city's historical lumber industry are never far from the trail or the bay. As you approach the city marina, about 3.4 miles from the southern endpoint, you'll spot lumber stacked to your left and a historical railcar on display to your right.

The trail has public access points for fishing, canoeing, paddleboarding, and kayaking. The public Del Norte Street Fishing Pier is just off the trail about 0.9 mile south of the city marina. While no fishing license is required at the time of publication, review the California Department of Fish and Wildlife's ocean-port fishing regulations at **rtc.li/ca-fish-wildlife.** To further explore the bay, head to the Eureka Slough Boat Ramp, just north of the city marina, for nonmotorized watercraft (learn more at **visiteureka.com**).

Tracing Eureka's waterfront, the trail offers access for fishing, boating, and paddle sports.   Brian Housh

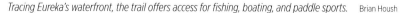

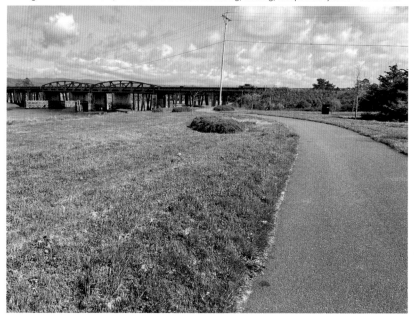

Near the trail's northern endpoint, you may either take a boardwalk extension to enjoy sweeping views of Humboldt Bay or follow a segment nearer the neighborhoods for access to the main trail boardwalk. Note that there is no parking area at the trail's northern endpoint on Tydd Street.

At the time of publication, a trail extension was underway to extend the southern endpoint an additional 1.1 miles from the Herrick Avenue Park & Ride to Tooby Road.

The Eureka Waterfront Trail is part of a larger project being developed by Humboldt County called the Humboldt Bay Trail, which will span 13 miles and connect Eureka to Arcata.

CONTACT ci.eureka.ca.gov/depts/pnr/trails

PARKING

Parking areas are located within Eureka and are listed from south to north. *Indicates that at least one accessible parking space is available.*

HERRICK AVENUE PARK & RIDE* Pound Road Herrick Ave., off US 101/Redwood Hwy. (40.7583, -124.1907); free parking.

POUND ROAD 0.1 mile west of US 101 (where Pound Road turns into Herrick Ave.) (40.7592, -124.1927).

HILFIKER LANE* Hilfiker Lane, 0.5 mile from the intersection with US 101/Redwood Hwy. (40.7685, -124.1964); the lot is at the end of Hilfiker Lane.

HIKSHARI' TRAILHEAD Hilfiker Lane, 0.2 mile west of US 101/Redwood Hwy. (40.7728, -124.1951); gravel parking lot.

TRUESDALE STREET TRAILHEAD* Truesdale St. and Christie St. (40.7760, -124.1938).

DEL NORTE PARK* W. Del Norte St., 0.1 mile west of Felt St. (40.7906, -124.1867); the parking lot is located at the west end of W. Del Norte St., near the Del Norte Street Fishing Pier.

SAMOA BRIDGE LAUNCHING FACILITY* Front St. and Waterfront Dr., on the underpass for CA 255/R St. (40.8076, -124.1537); includes trailered boat area.

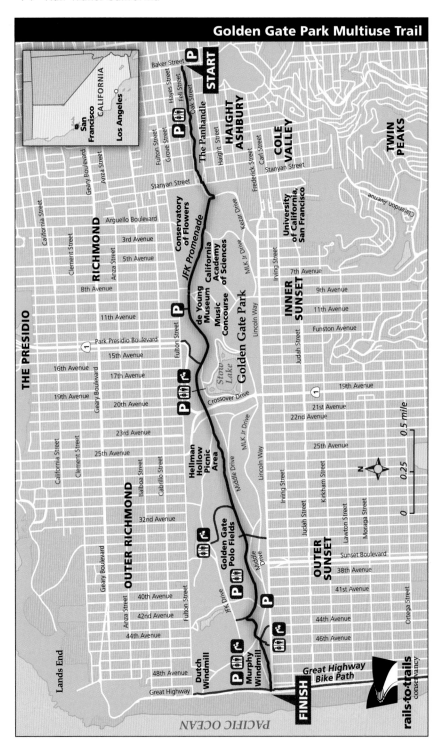

Golden Gate Park Multiuse Trail

CALIFORNIA

San Francisco

CALIFORNIA

Los Angeles

START

Baker Street

Hayes Street

Fell Street

Oak Street

The Panhandle

HAIGHT ASHBURY

Fulton Street

Grove Street

Haight Street

Frederick Street

Carl Street

COLE VALLEY

Stanyan Street

Stanyan Street

TWIN PEAKS

Clarendon Avenue

Geary Boulevard

Anza Street

California Street

Clement Street

Arguello Boulevard

RICHMOND

3rd Avenue

5th Avenue

Anza Street

8th Avenue

Conservatory of Flowers

JFK Promenade

California Academy of Sciences

Kezar Drive

MLK Jr Drive

University of California, San Francisco

7th Avenue

Irving Street

9th Avenue

11th Avenue

INNER SUNSET

Funston Avenue

THE PRESIDIO

11th Avenue

Park Presidio Boulevard

15th Avenue

16th Avenue

17th Avenue

19th Avenue

20th Avenue

Geary Boulevard

de Young Museum

Music Concourse

Golden Gate Park

Stow Lake

Fulton Street

Crossover Drive

Lincoln Way

Judah Street

19th Avenue

21st Avenue

22nd Avenue

23rd Avenue

25th Avenue

California Street

Clement Street

Balboa Street

Cabrillo Street

Hellman Hollow Picnic Area

MLK Jr Drive

Middle Drive

Lincoln Way

25th Avenue

Irving Street

Judah Street

Kirkham Street

Lawton Street

Moraga Street

N

0.5 mile

0.25

0

32nd Avenue

OUTER RICHMOND

Geary Boulevard

40th Avenue

42nd Avenue

44th Avenue

Anza Street

Fulton Street

JFK Drive

Golden Gate Polo Fields

Middle Drive

Sunset Boulevard

OUTER SUNSET

38th Avenue

41st Avenue

44th Avenue

46th Avenue

Ortega Street

Lands End

48th Avenue

Dutch Windmill

Murphy Windmill

Great Highway

FINISH

Great Highway Bike Path

PACIFIC OCEAN

rails-to-trails
conservancy

At more than 1,000 acres, San Francisco's Golden Gate Park is one of the nation's top urban green spaces, welcoming 24 million visitors each year. Several roadways are either closed to vehicles or have very low traffic—and in 2022, the eastern portion of JFK Drive was permanently closed to vehicles, transforming one of the city's most dangerous stretches of road into a wide public pathway for rolling and strolling to the park's most popular attractions. These low-stress roadways string together a virtually car-free route that follows the length of the park, giving visitors access to picnic areas, restrooms, and other amenities.

This route is part of a developing 2,600-miles-plus Bay Area regional trail network being spearheaded by the Bay Area Trails Collaborative (**railstotrails.org/bay-area**) and Rails-to-Trails Conservancy as a TrailNation™ project to increase safe walking, biking, and trail access for millions of Bay Area residents.

Begin your journey on the far east side of Golden Gate Park, where a popular multiuse pathway winds through

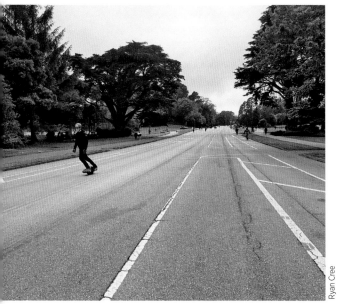

Ryan Cree

Within Golden Gate Park, a closed-to-vehicles portion of JFK Drive now serves as a public pathway.

County
San Francisco

Endpoints
Fell St. and Baker St.;
Martin Luther King Jr. Dr.,
250 feet east of the Great
Hwy. and Lincoln Way
intersection

Mileage
3.9

Type
Greenway/Non-Rail-Trail

Roughness Rating
1

Surface
Asphalt

the narrowest portion of the park, known as The Panhandle. Here, many gather to stroll along the various paths, play at the playgrounds and basketball court, or simply enjoy the open green space under the shade of trees. The pathway starts at the northeast corner of the park at the intersection of Fell Street and Baker Street. Plentiful street parking is available along the perimeter of the park.

The Panhandle and the pathway come to an end at Stanyan Street. Turn right to access the Fell Street bike lane on the north side of the street. As you cross Stanyan, Fell Street becomes John F. Kennedy Drive (JFK Drive) and merges into the main section of Golden Gate Park. Here, JFK Drive becomes the newly opened, car-free JFK Promenade.

For the next 1.4 miles, the expanse of JFK Promenade provides a safe and leisurely way to access the park's major attractions. Soon after entering the park, the Conservatory of Flowers will be on your right. The de Young Museum, showcasing fine art and a sculpture garden, and the California Academy of Sciences will be farther down on the left.

Spanning 1,000 acres, Golden Gate Park offers expansive green space in the heart of San Francisco.
TrailLink user ramoshunter933

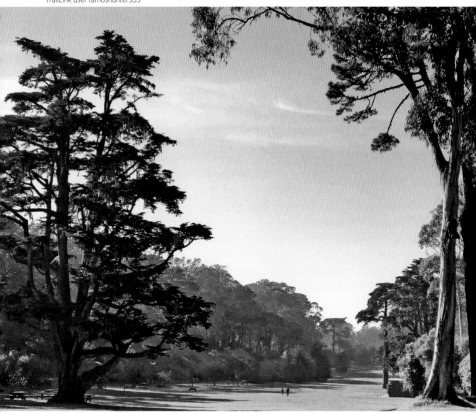

Use caution after passing under Crossover Drive, as cars are present here on JFK Drive and Transverse Road. Turn left on Transverse Road and then take an immediate right onto Overlook Drive. This tree-lined section is once again car-free, traveling past the wide grassy lawn of Hellman Hollow Picnic Area. Overlook Drive merges with the lightly trafficked Middle Drive as you travel downhill toward the polo fields (on the right).

The pathway ends on Martin Luther King Jr. Drive near the intersection of Great Highway and Lincoln Way, just past the Murphy Windmill, once one of the largest of its kind outside the Netherlands. The windmill, along with the Dutch Windmill in the northwestern corner of the park, pumped water during the early 20th century to transform the area's former sand dunes into the lush green park you see today.

Take a right onto Lincoln Way to connect to the Great Highway Bike Path, which parallels Ocean Beach for spectacular views of the Pacific Ocean.

CONTACT rtc.li/san-francisco-parks

PARKING

Parking areas are located within San Francisco and are listed from east to west. Select parking areas for the trail are listed below. For a detailed list of parking areas and other waypoints, go to **TrailLink.com™**. *Indicates that at least one accessible parking space is available.*

THE PANHANDLE Parking is available along Baker St., between Oak St. and Fell St., on the eastern end of Golden Gate Park known as The Panhandle (37.7732, -122.4409).

STOW LAKE BOATHOUSE* 50 Stow Lake Dr. (37.7708, -122.4772).

GOLDEN GATE PARK POLO FIELDS* On the southwestern end of the field off Middle Dr., 0.1 mile north of Martin Luther King Jr. Dr. (37.7667, -122.4948).

CHAIN OF LAKES MEADOW Chain of Lakes Dr., 500 feet north of Martin Luther King Jr. Dr. (37.7659, -122.4999).

GREAT HIGHWAY PARKING* Great Hwy., between Lincoln Way and John F. Kennedy Dr. (37.7676, -122.5108).

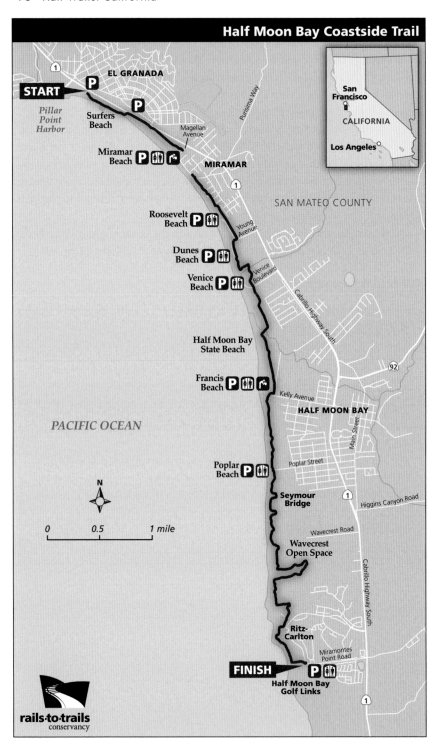

Half Moon Bay Coastside Trail

San Francisco

CALIFORNIA

Los Angeles

START

Pillar
Point
Harbor

EL GRANADA

Surfers
Beach

Miramar
Beach

MIRAMAR

Magellan
Avenue

Purisima Way

SAN MATEO COUNTY

Roosevelt
Beach

Young
Avenue

Dunes
Beach

Venice
Boulevard

Venice
Beach

Cabrillo Highway South

Half Moon Bay
State Beach

Francis
Beach

Kelly Avenue

HALF MOON BAY

PACIFIC OCEAN

Main Street

Poplar
Beach

Poplar Street

Seymour
Bridge

Higgins Canyon Road

N

0   0.5   1 mile

Wavecrest Road

Wavecrest
Open Space

Cabrillo Highway South

Ritz-
Carlton

Miramontes
Point Road

FINISH

Half Moon Bay
Golf Links

rails·to·trails
conservancy

Visitors to the Half Moon Bay Coastside Trail, which traces a bluff overlooking the Pacific Ocean, will get a front-row seat to the sight of waves crashing onto the beach, whales migrating way out at sea, or a heartwarming sunset at the end of the day. Spanning 7.5 miles, it runs the length of Half Moon Bay State Beach and a little beyond—from Pillar Point Harbor in El Granada to the Half Moon Bay Golf Links.

The rail-trail roughly follows the corridor of the short-lived Ocean Shore Railroad, which launched shortly before the 1906 San Francisco earthquake. Although passengers used the railroad to visit the beaches, it went out of business in 1920 as farmers came to rely on trucks to get their produce to market.

The state park offers parking, picnicking, fishing, and camping, and visitors are encouraged to arrive early on weekends. Facilities are wheelchair accessible, right down

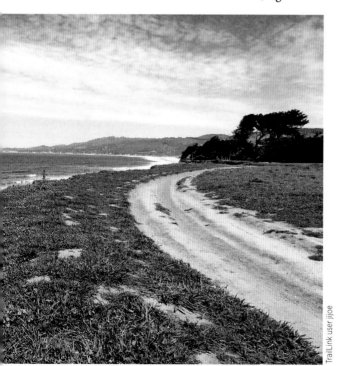

The Coastside Trail runs the length of Half Moon Bay State Beach.

TrailLink user jijoe

County
San Mateo

Endpoints
Pillar Point Harbor
Blvd., 0.3 mile east of
Capistrano Road
(El Granada); Miramontes
Point Road, 0.6 mile
west of Cabrillo Hwy./
CA 1 (Half Moon Bay)

Mileage
7.5

Type
Rail-Trail

Roughness Rating
1

Surface
Asphalt

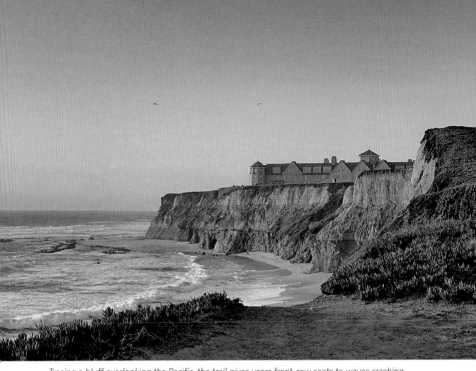

Tracing a bluff overlooking the Pacific, the trail gives users front-row seats to waves crashing onto the beach. TrailLink user khoaduynguyen

to the availability of wheelchairs with balloon-style wheels for crossing the sand at Francis Beach. There's access from the trail to all the popular beaches along this stretch. Sunbathing is welcome, but swimming is discouraged due to dangerous currents and the absence of lifeguards.

Starting at Pillar Point Harbor in El Granada, visitors will quickly be aware of another popular diversion: surfing. After passing a forest of sailboat masts at the marina, you'll cross the jetty to Surfers Beach, which experiences good waves under the right conditions. (About 2 miles northwest is world-renowned Mavericks Beach, where 15- to 30-foot waves challenge surfers.)

Less than a mile from the harbor, the trail veers away from Cabrillo Highway/CA 1. At 1 mile, the trail ends at Magellan Avenue but resumes in 0.3 mile at Miramar Beach. To pick up the trail again, take a right on Magellan Avenue, then take your first left on Mirada Road, which ends at the beach. Here the trail follows the bluff past a series of beaches—Roosevelt, Dunes, and Venice—and park entrances at Young Avenue and Venice Boulevard.

The main park entrance and visitor center (open weekends only) is at Francis Beach at the end of Kelly Avenue, 2.4 miles from Miramar Beach. Here you'll find camping, picnicking, and the start of an equestrian trail that is separated from the Coastside Trail by a split-rail fence and runs about a mile south to

Poplar Beach. If you stray off the Coastside Trail onto the beach, stay a safe distance from temporary fencing that protects the nesting areas of the tiny western snowy plover, a threatened species.

The trail crosses the Seymour Bridge over a drainage in 1.1 miles. The Monterey pines and eucalyptus trees here offer some rare shade along the route. For the next 2.7 miles, the trail passes through wildlife and bird habitat at the Wavecrest Open Space before ending at the Half Moon Bay Golf Links.

The paved pathway is also a segment of the California Coastal Trail, a network of bicycling and hiking trails that, when complete, will stretch along the coastline for 1,230 miles from Oregon to the Mexican border. Another segment of the California Coastal Trail, the Cowell-Purisima Trail (see page 49), begins about a mile south.

Caution: Due to the 2022–2023 storms, erosion has occurred along the Half Moon Bay Coastside Trail. As improvements are ongoing, visitors are encouraged to sign up for the City of Half Moon Bay's e-news bulletin for updates at **rtc.li/half-moon-bay.**

CONTACT **parks.ca.gov/?page_id=531**

PARKING

Parking areas are listed from north to south. *Indicates that at least one accessible parking space is available.*

EL GRANADA* Pillar Point Launch Ramp, 67173 Pillar Point Harbor Blvd., 450 feet east of Capistrano Road (37.5040, -122.4807).

EL GRANADA Magellan Ave., 300 feet west of Cabrillo Hwy./CA 1 (37.4967, -122.4616); limited parking.

HALF MOON BAY* Roosevelt Beach, Entrance at Young Ave., 0.3 mile west of Cabrillo Hwy./CA 1, then north 0.2 mile (37.4884, -122.4549).

HALF MOON BAY* Dunes Beach, Entrance at Young Ave., 0.3 mile west of Cabrillo Hwy./CA 1, then south 350 feet (37.4847, -122.4527).

HALF MOON BAY* Venice Beach, 400 Venice Blvd., 0.3 mile west of Cabrillo Hwy./CA 1 (37.4791, -122.4491).

HALF MOON BAY* Francis Beach, 440 Balboa Blvd. (37.4668, -122.4449).

HALF MOON BAY* Poplar Beach, Poplar St., 0.2 mile west of Railroad Ave. (37.4552, -122.4436).

HALF MOON BAY* Manhattan Beach, 1001 Miramontes Point Road (37.4304, -122.4371).

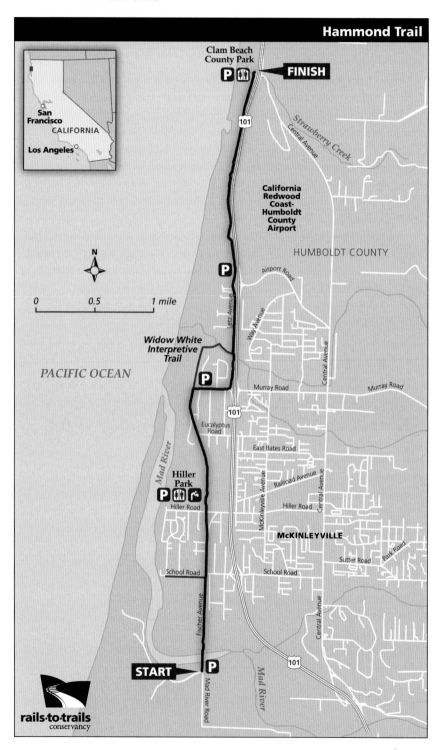

Hammond Trail

Clam Beach County Park

FINISH

101

Strawberry Creek

Central Avenue

California Redwood Coast-Humboldt County Airport

HUMBOLDT COUNTY

San Francisco

CALIFORNIA

Los Angeles

N

Airport Road

Letz Avenue

Way Avenue

Central Avenue

0   0.5   1 mile

Widow White Interpretive Trail

Murray Road   Murray Road

PACIFIC OCEAN

101

Eucalyptus Road

East Bates Road

McKinleyville Avenue

Railroad Avenue

Central Avenue

Mad River

Hiller Park

Hiller Road

Hiller Road

McKINLEYVILLE

Sutter Road

Park Road

School Road   School Road

Fischer Avenue

Central Avenue

START

101

Mad River

Mad River Road

rails·to·trails
conservancy

The Hammond Trail pays homage to the Redwood Coast's timber industry. Named for a major local lumber company, the asphalt, gravel, and dirt trail follows the route of a former railroad that hauled timber out of the expansive Humboldt County redwood forests to the Hammond Redwood Co. in Samoa on Humboldt Bay, a few miles south of where the trail ends today.

Along the 5.5-mile route, you'll pass through farmland and forested bluffs overlooking the Mad River, as well as beach-access points. The trail is a segment of the California Coastal Trail, a network of bicycling and hiking trails that, when complete, will stretch along the coastline for 1,230 miles from Oregon to the Mexican border.

Hammond Lumber Company got its start in 1863 and eventually gained control of the Humboldt Northern Railroad, which ran between Humboldt Bay in the south and the company town of Crannell in the north. The company stopped operating the railroad in the 1950s, and the first segment of the Hammond Trail opened in 1983.

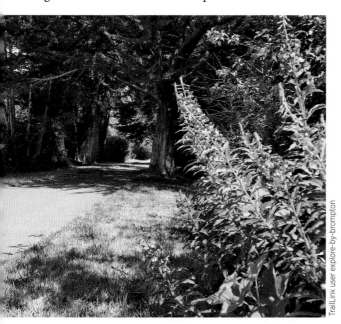

Native plants, like this fireweed with vibrant magenta flowers, line the path.

TrailLink user explore-by-brompton

County
Humboldt

Endpoints
Mad River Bridge on Mad River Road, 1.7 miles from the intersection with Miller Lane (Arcata); Clam Beach County Park at Clam Beach Dr., about 300 feet from US 101 Business (McKinleyville)

Mileage
5.5

Type
Rail-Trail

Roughness Rating
2

Surface
Asphalt, Gravel, Dirt

The trail starts in the south at a trestle crossing over the Mad River. According to local lore, the river earned its name during an 1849 expedition when a surveyor launched into a memorable and expletive-filled tirade when his fellow explorers began crossing the river in their canoes without him.

The trestle itself is due for replacement. The original span, a covered bridge built in 1905, was replaced in 1941 by a bridge relocated from Washington state and reassembled here. Today the bridge provides a scenic overlook of the area and the opportunity to see marine mammals, such as seals and sea otters. Many bird species, including cormorants, grebes, herons, ducks, and Aleutian geese, endangered until recently, also frequent the area.

Crossing the bridge, you'll share the road with lightly used Fischer Avenue for about a half mile to a short climb into the community of McKinleyville. You'll find a grocery at School Road, where a 0.3-mile spur trail to the left leads you to within sight of the Mad River. Continuing north on the Hammond Trail, you'll arrive at Hiller Park in 0.7 mile. Here, about 1.5 miles of paths meander

The Hammond Trail's northern portion offers ocean views and access to Clam Beach County Park.
TrailLink user majipoor

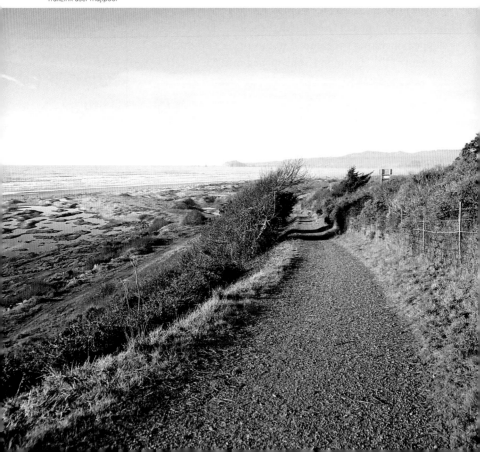

through native coastal trees to a bluff overlooking the Mad River and a long sand spit separating it from the ocean beyond.

Leaving the parking lot at Hiller Park, the trail follows a woodsy corridor north 0.9 mile to a trail split. The Hammond Trail, which travels the paved right fork—traces Murray Road east on a 0.3-mile bike lane, then heads north alongside US 101/Redwood Highway. The gravel left fork overlooks the Mad River and ocean along a wooded bluff before turning inland back to the Hammond Trail via the hiker-only Widow White Interpretive Trail. Bicyclists and horseback riders can use the spur to Sandpointe Drive to get back to Murray Road.

The remaining 2.4 miles of trail are both paved and dirt as the route travels along the highway—and a half mile on Letz Avenue—to Clam Beach County Park, which is popular for beachcombing, horseback riding, and, of course, clamming. You'll also find beach campsites and restrooms. The park is connected to the north with Little River State Beach to create a 5-mile stretch of beach.

CONTACT **humboldtgov.org/2761/hammond-trail**

PARKING

Parking areas are listed from south to north. *Indicates that at least one accessible parking space is available.*

ARCATA* Hammond Trail Trailhead, 789 Mad River Road (40.9229, -124.1202).

MCKINLEYVILLE* Hiller Park, 300 feet north of the intersection of Hiller Road and Fischer Ave. (40.9429, -124.1203).

MCKINLEYVILLE* Murray Road and Kelly Ave. (40.9563, -124.1218).

MCKINLEYVILLE* 3451 Letz Ave. (40.9710, -124.1166).

MCKINLEYVILLE* Clam Beach County Park, 1100 Clam Beach Dr. (40.9942, -124.1141).

Humboldt Bay Trail North

Foster Avenue

Grant Avenue

101

START

Foster Avenue

17th Street

Shay Park

Larson Park

Janes Road

16th Street

15th Street

13th Street

14th Street

Cal Poly Humboldt

M Street

I Street

11th Street

E Street

11th Street

Union Street

Q Street

N Street

9th Street

D Street

C Street

Arcata Community Forest

11th Street

ARCATA

K Street

Arcata Plaza

7th Street

255

Samoa Boulevard

L Street

H Street

A Street

South Street

4th Street

Arcata Sports Complex

Bayside Road

Arcata Marsh & Wildlife Sanctuary

South G Street

F Street

Klopp Lake

South G Street

101

Old Arcata Road

Buttermilk Lane

HUMBOLDT COUNTY

Arcata Bay

Redwood Highway

N

0   0.25   0.5 mile

Old Arcata Road

Bayside Cutoff

FINISH

101

San Francisco

CALIFORNIA

Los Angeles

rails·to·trails
conservancy

The Humboldt Bay Trail North runs from central Arcata, near the campus of Cal Poly Humboldt, through town, and then meanders through the lush Arcata Marsh & Wildlife Sanctuary. An extension of the flat, paved trail continues south along Arcata Bay, a northern arm of Humboldt Bay. The trail is a segment of the developing California Coastal Trail, a network of bicycling and hiking trails that, when complete, will stretch along the coastline for 1,230 miles from Oregon to the Mexican border.

The route roughly follows the Humboldt County section of the Northwestern Pacific Railroad, which hauled timber from the coastal forests in the 19th and 20th centuries. Visitors can still see the rusting rails in several locations along the route.

The trail begins near the Arcata Skate Park and high school sports fields in the north, just across US 101/Redwood Highway from the college campus. It heads west along Foster Avenue before turning south along Alliance

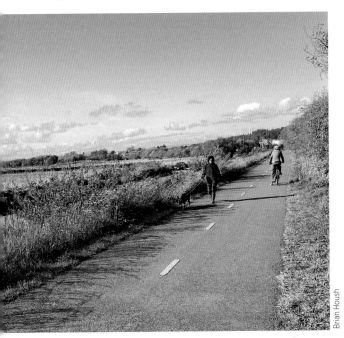

Brian Housh

The southern end of the trail follows Arcata Bay, a northern arm of Humboldt Bay.

County
Humboldt

Endpoints
Traffic circle at Foster Ave. and Sunset Ave. (Arcata); US 101/ Redwood Hwy., 0.2 mile south of Bayside Cutoff (Arcata)

Mileage
4.5

Type
Rail-Trail

Roughness Rating
1

Surface
Asphalt

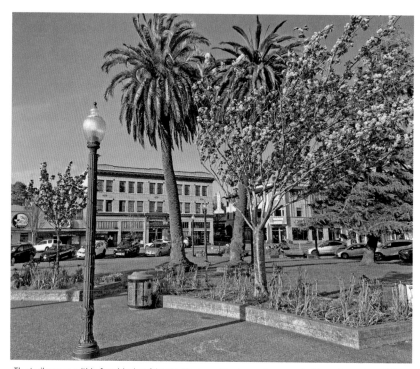

The trail passes within four blocks of Arcata Plaza, a gathering spot surrounded by restaurants and shops.
Brian Housh

Road and L Street in Shay Park. Traversing the western side of Arcata's compact, lively downtown, the trail passes within four blocks of Arcata Plaza, a community gathering spot surrounded by restaurants and shops. A painted design on the pavement of Ninth Street leads the way to an interesting array of murals rendered throughout downtown.

Crossing busy Samoa Boulevard in 1.3 miles, the trail leaves the urban landscape and enters a different environment: the 307-acre Arcata Marsh and Wildlife Sanctuary. Just off Arcata Bay, this scenic, marshy area of lush vegetation draws bird-watchers and features several miles of hiking paths and an interpretive center.

The southern portion of the trail presents another change as it runs through tidal mudflats of Arcata Bay, buffered by brush and small trees that hide the old railroad tracks. US 101 parallels the trail on its inland side, interrupting the natural atmosphere with high-speed traffic.

Currently, the trail ends abruptly along US 101, 0.2 mile south of Bayside Cutoff at the Arcata city limits. Consider starting your visit at another access point farther north, as there is no parking or safe place to pull over at the southern endpoint, and accessing it by bike or foot involves a dangerous crossing.

This segment is the latest phase in an ongoing rail-trail project to connect central Arcata with Eureka (to the south) for a total distance of 14 miles. In 2019, the state allocated construction funding to close the 4-mile gap between the Humboldt Bay Trail North and the Eureka Waterfront Trail (see page 71), with work slated to begin in 2023 and end in 2024.

CONTACT rtc.li/humboldt-bay-trail-north

PARKING

Parking areas are located within Arcata and are listed from north to south. *Indicates that at least one accessible parking space is available.*

LARSON PARK*: Eye St., between Jay St. and Todd Ct. (40.8808, -124.0835). This lot is less than 0.2 mile away from the northern endpoint. From the lot, access the trail by heading west on Eye St. for 300 feet, and then south (left) onto Jay St. for 0.1 mile. The trailhead is on the other side of the traffic circle.

ARCATA MARSH & WILDLIFE SANCTUARY S. I St., 0.3 mile southwest of CA 255/Samoa Blvd. (40.8616, -124.0925).

ARCATA MARSH & WILDLIFE SANCTUARY S. I St., 0.5 mile southwest of CA 225/Samoa Blvd. (40.8587, -124.0950).

ARCATA MARSH & WILDLIFE SANCTUARY S. I St., 1 mile southwest of CA 225/Samoa Blvd. (40.8558, -124.0981).

ARCATA CITY YARD* 600 S. G St., 0.4 mile northwest of southbound Exit 712 on US 101/ Redwood Hwy. (40.8554, -124.0892); park outside the fence.

On-street parking is available on Foster Ave. near Shay Park, between Western Ave. and Eastern Ave. (40.8793, -124.0904).

Humbug-Willow Creek Trail

rails·to·trails
conservancy

Sophia Parkway

East Natoma Street

Golf Links Drive

Broadstone Parkway

East Natoma

East Natoma Street

Green Valley Road

Folsom Point State Park

Elvie Perazzo Briggs Park

Folsom Lake

START

Econome Family Park

Philip C. Cohn Park

Silberhorn Drive

SACRAMENTO COUNTY

East Bidwell Street

Oak Avenue Parkway

N

1 mile

0.5

0

Oak Avenue Parkway

Blue Ravine Road

Creekside Drive

Cummings Family Skate & Bike Park

Humbug Creek

Willow Creek

Riley Street

Iron Point Road

Oak Parkway Trail

Johnny Cash Trail

Folsom State Prison

East Bidwell Street

Jim Konopka Volunteer Bridge

Amos P. Catlin Park

Russi Road

Prairie City Road

Natoma Street

Riley Street

Sutter Street

Sibley Street

FOLSOM

Glen Station Park & Ride

Glen Drive

Coolidge Dr

Folsom Boulevard

Blue Ravine Road

Natoma Station Drive

FINISH

Folsom-Auburn Road

Folsom Parkway Rail Trail

American River Parkway (Jedediah Smith Memorial Trail)

Lake Natoma

Willow Creek Recreation Area

Folsom Blvd

CALIFORNIA

San Francisco

Los Angeles

The Humbug–Willow Creek Trail shows community at its best, offering plenty of sights, sounds, and activities as it snakes through the city of Folsom. The trail is embedded within a greenbelt that runs through the heart of the city, preserving natural habitats while providing an easily accessible escape from city life. Segments of the trail are set in open, rolling grasslands; farther southwest, the path provides a vantage point from which to observe the colorfully diverse fauna and flora of wetland ponds. Railroad tracks emerge seemingly out of nowhere and then disappear behind trees.

There are dozens of places—including many spurs—to access the trail. Steeper sections are found near the southern endpoint, near Folsom Boulevard and Lake Natoma. For details on wheelchair-accessible sections of the trail, reach out to the Friends of Folsom Parkways at **enjoyfolsomtrails.org.** The main spines generally follow Humbug and Willow Creeks, but the spurs, curves, and intersections make it easy to get turned around, so you might want to pack a map.

County
Sacramento

Endpoints
Econome Family Park, Blue Ravine Road and Parkway Dr. (Folsom); Creekside Dr., 0.1 mile northeast of E. Bidwell St. (Folsom); E. Bidwell St., 0.1 mile southeast of Creekside Dr. (Folsom); Folsom Pkwy. Rail Trail, 500 feet southeast of Folsom Blvd. and Parkshore Dr. (Folsom); Folsom Blvd. and Woodmere Road (Folsom); Willow Creek Recreation Area at Folsom Blvd., near Natoma Station Dr. (Folsom)

Mileage
15

Type
Greenway/Non-Rail-Trail, Rail-with-Trail

Roughness Rating
1

Surface
Asphalt, Boardwalk

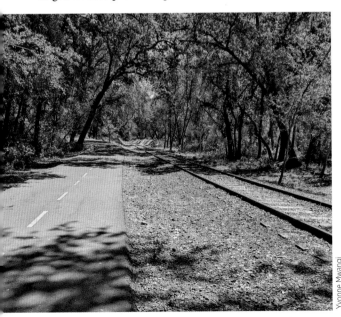

Yvonne Mwangi

Largely tucked into the trees, the trail offers a natural oasis in Folsom.

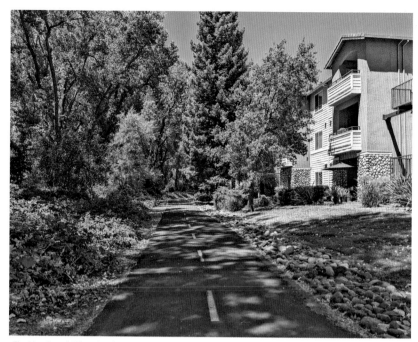

The Humbug–Willow Creek Trail is embedded within a greenbelt that runs through the heart of Folsom.
Yvonne Mwangi

Begin at Parkway Drive at Econome Family Park, one of several well-maintained parks through which the trail threads. North of the park is a shopping center if you need to refuel upon your return. Heading east from the park, the winding trail spits into several branches. Consult your map or GPS app to navigate southwest toward Phillip C. Cohn Park, the next park in the route along the Humbug Creek branch.

At Oak Avenue Parkway, those following Humbug Creek can take the crosswalk at Blue Raven Road to the north or Creekside Drive to the south. Those on the Willow Creek branch can take the midblock signalized crossing. In a commercial corridor at East Bidwell Street, a pedestrian bridge delivers users safely across. Around mile 3.8 is the 300-foot, curving wooden Jim Konopka Volunteer Bridge, named for Folsom's senior trail planner and architect of the city's recreational pathway system, who led a team of 49 volunteers to complete the bridge over 12 weekends.

Near the trail's southern end, you'll use tunnels to pass beneath city streets. There are also some segments adjacent to fast-moving traffic on Blue Ravine Road. The two branches of the trail meet at Riley Street and continue as one toward Folsom Boulevard, meeting the 2.9-mile Folsom Parkway Rail Trail, which leads to Historic Folsom, a good place to stop and enjoy one of many nice eateries. Cross Folsom Boulevard at Parkshore Drive and head 0.2 mile south using the on-street bike lane or sidewalk to travel to Woodmere Road, where you can pick up the trail (and nature) again. The trail follows Willow Creek as it meanders to Lake Natoma at the Willow Creek Recreation Area.

The trail also connects to the 3.2-mile Johnny Cash Trail and the 32-mile American River Parkway (Jedediah Smith Memorial Trail; see page 13), stretching from Folsom Lake south to Sacramento.

CONTACT rtc.li/humbug-willow-creek-trail

PARKING

Parking areas are located within Folsom and are listed from northeast to southwest. *Indicates that at least one accessible parking space is available.*

ELVIE PERAZZO BRIGGS PARK* Manseau Dr. and Arrowsmith Dr. (38.6885, -121.1256); there is no direct trail access, but users can cross Blue Ravine Road to reach Econome Family Park.

ECONOME FAMILY PARK* Blue Ravine Road and Parkway Dr. (38.6873, -121.1227).

PHILLIP C. COHN PARK* Prewett Dr., north of N. Lexington Dr. (38.6751, -121.1258); across from Oak Chan Elementary School.

CUMMINGS FAMILY SKATE & BIKE PARK* Oak Avenue Pkwy. and Creekside Dr. (38.6735, -121.1368).

AMOS P. CATLIN PARK Russi Road near Grover Road (38.6546, -121.1571).

GLENN STATION PARK & RIDE* Glenn Dr. and Coolidge Dr. (38.6633, -121.1825).

AMERICAN RIVER PARKWAY TRAILHEAD* Parkshore Dr., 0.1 mile west of Folsom Blvd. (38.6589, -121.1853).

WILLOW CREEK RECREATION AREA* Folsom Blvd., 0.7 mile southwest of Blue Ravine Road (38.6485, -121.1899). Day-use parking fees apply; learn more at: **rtc.li/ca-parks-rec.**

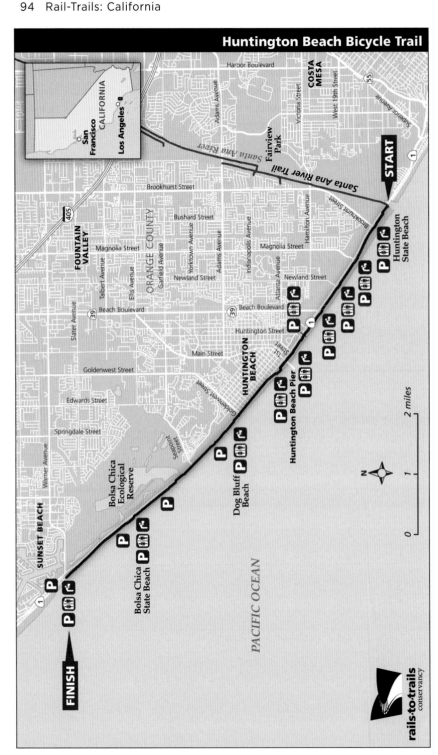

Huntington Beach Bicycle Trail

The Huntington Beach Bicycle Trail fulfills visitors' every expectation about what they'll find in a town dubbed Surf City USA. Following the Pacific Coast for its entire 8.3 miles, the trail provides plenty of opportunities to catch some rays, join a pickup game of beach volleyball, and live your California fantasy.

The fully paved trail is part of the California Coastal Trail, a developing network that, when complete, will stretch for 1,230 miles from Oregon to the Mexican border. At the southeast end, the Huntington Beach Bicycle Trail connects to the Santa Ana River Trail (see page 215), which follows that river inland some 50 miles. The transition between the two is seamless.

For those arriving by car, the first parking area in the south is at Brookhurst Street, about 0.4 mile northwest of the trail's endpoint. Ample parking for the beach is provided along almost the entire length of the trail, although fees are charged. There also are dozens of restrooms and water fountains.

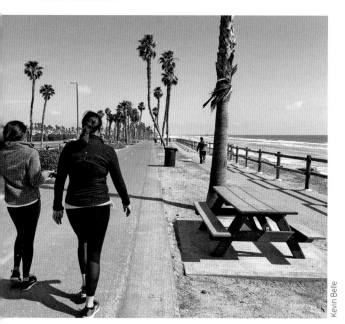

Kevin Belle

With two state beaches and miles of coastline, this is a genuine Southern California experience.

County
Orange

Endpoints
Santa Ana River Trail at CA 1/Pacific Coast Hwy., 0.4 mile south of Brookhurst St. (Huntington Beach); Sunset Beach at Warner Ave. and N. Pacific Ave. (Huntington Beach)

Mileage
8.3

Type
Greenway/Non-Rail-Trail

Roughness Rating
1

Surface
Asphalt, Concrete

Concessions, such as restaurants, surf shops, and bike rentals, are located along the trail as well. They're sparsely placed at first, but they get more frequent as you head north. The trail can get crowded near the denser concession areas; make sure to slow down to give everyone space, and take the time to soak in the laid-back Huntington Beach vibe.

About 3 miles north of the Santa Ana River is the Huntington Beach Pier, jutting 1,800 feet into the ocean and practically demanding that you take a brief detour. (Note that the pier passes over the trail, and bicycles are not allowed on the pier.) If you're lucky, you might get to see the filming of a TV show or movie around this iconic spot. The pier is also popular with anglers looking to reel in a nice perch, a mackerel, or even a shark. A fishing permit is not required on the public pier, unlike other places in and around Huntington Beach.

The people-watching alone is worth a visit to this trail. From in-line skaters and skateboarders to weight lifters and sunbathers, the trail attracts a diverse and unique crowd. Huntington Beach declares itself Surf City USA, and you can quickly tell why when you see the number of wet suit–clad surfers carrying their boards to and from the coastline.

About 4 miles north of the pier, visitors will travel through Bolsa Chica State Park, which provides RV spots and fire rings for those wishing to linger for the beautiful beach sunsets. Across the Pacific Coast Highway is Bolsa Chica Ecological Reserve, a coastal habitat for more than 200 species of shorebirds.

The trail ends another 1.5 miles north at Warner Avenue by Sunset Beach.

CONTACT surfcityusa.com/things-to-do/activities/biking

PARKING

Parking areas are located within Huntington Beach and are listed from south to north. Be prepared to pay a fee. Select parking areas for the trail are listed below. For a detailed list of parking areas and other waypoints, go to **TrailLink.com**™. *Indicates that at least one accessible parking space is available.*

HUNTINGTON STATE BEACH* CA 1/E. Pacific Coast Hwy., at Brookhurst St. (33.6339, -117.9626).

HUNTINGTON STATE BEACH* CA 1/E. Pacific Coast Hwy., at Magnolia St. (33.6387, -117.9720).

HUNTINGTON STATE BEACH* CA 1/E. Pacific Coast Hwy., at Newland St. (33.6430, -117.9796).

HUNTINGTON STATE BEACH* CA 1/E. Pacific Coast Hwy. at Beach Blvd. (33.6471, -117.9866).

HUNTINGTON CITY BEACH* CA 1/ E. Pacific Coast Hwy. at Huntington St. (33.6525, -117.9956).

HUNTINGTON CITY BEACH* CA 1/ E. Pacific Coast Hwy. at First. St. (33.6549, -117.9993).

HUNTINGTON CITY BEACH* CA 1/ E. Pacific Coast Hwy. at Sixth St. (33.6583, -118.0042).

DOG BEACH BLUFF* CA 1/E. Pacific Coast Hwy., between Seapoint St. and Goldenwest St. (33.6716, -118.0224).

BOLSA CHICA STATE BEACH* CA 1/E. Pacific Coast Hwy., between Seapoint St. and Warner Ave. (33.6939, -118.0461).

SUNSET BEACH* N. Pacific Ave. and Warner Ave. (33.7123, -118.0646).

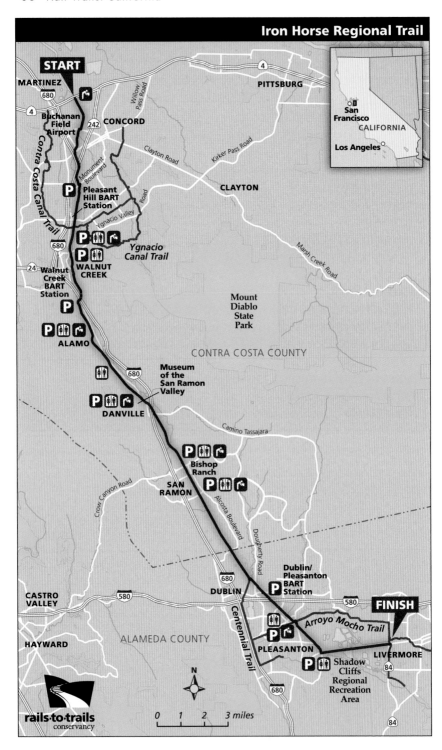

Iron Horse Regional Trail

START

MARTINEZ

680

4

Buchanan Field Airport

242 CONCORD

Willow Pass Road

PITTSBURG

4

San Francisco

CALIFORNIA

Los Angeles

Contra Costa Canal Trail

Clayton Road

Kirker Pass Road

CLAYTON

Monument Boulevard

P Pleasant Hill BART Station

Ygnacio Valley Road

680

P

P WALNUT CREEK

Ygnacio Canal Trail

24 Walnut Creek BART Station

Marsh Creek Road

P

P ALAMO

Mount Diablo State Park

CONTRA COSTA COUNTY

680 Museum of the San Ramon Valley

P DANVILLE

Camino Tassajara

P Bishop Ranch

SAN RAMON

P

Crow Canyon Road

Alcosta Boulevard

Dougherty Road

Dublin/ Pleasanton BART Station P

CASTRO VALLEY

580

DUBLIN

580 FINISH

HAYWARD

ALAMEDA COUNTY

Centennial Trail

P

PLEASANTON

Arroyo Mocho Trail

LIVERMORE

84

P Shadow Cliffs Regional Recreation Area

680

84

N

0 1 2 3 miles

rails·to·trails
conservancy

unning north–south though San Francisco's East Bay region, the popular Iron Horse Regional Trail—whose very name conjures its important railroad history—follows the old Southern Pacific rail corridor, created in 1891. After the tracks fell into disuse in the late 1970s, the corridor was purchased by Alameda and Contra Costa Counties. Spanning 32 miles, it's one of the longest rail-trails in California.

The route roughly parallels I-680 and is heavily used for both recreation and commuting, connecting kids to schools, commuters to business centers, and residents to parks and other amenities. It connects nine cities and several Bay Area Rapid Transit (BART) stations, making it easily accessible without a car. Horseback riding opportunities vary by city; equestrians can contact the East Bay Regional Park District for more information. This trail

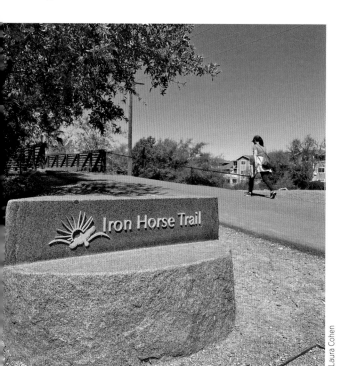

Running between Concord and Livermore, the trail offers access to neighborhoods, retail centers, parks, and transportation options.

Laura Cohen

Counties
Alameda, Contra Costa

Endpoints
Marsh Dr., 0.1 mile west of Solano Way (Concord); Stanley Blvd. and Isabel Ave. (Livermore)

Mileage
32

Type
Rail-Trail

Roughness Rating
1

Surface
Asphalt

is part of a developing 2,600-miles-plus Bay Area regional trail network being spearheaded by the Bay Area Trails Collaborative (**railstotrails.org/bay-area**) and Rails-to-Trails Conservancy as a TrailNation™ project to increase safe walking, biking, and trail access for millions of Bay Area residents.

At the northern end, the trail begins just south of CA 4, near the northeast corner of Buchanan Field Airport in Concord. Heading south, the trail hugs Walnut Creek for about 3.5 miles, providing good opportunities to see ducks, geese, egrets, and other birds. It diverges from the creek as it crosses Monument Boulevard in Pleasant Hill to connect with the Pleasant Hill BART station.

Continuing south from the station, the area becomes more urban, passing near downtown Walnut Creek and then gliding over two bridges for bicyclists and pedestrians that span Treat Boulevard and Ygnacio Valley Road. Between the two bridges, you'll cross the Contra Costa Canal Regional Trail (see page 45). You can access the Walnut Creek BART station by taking Ygnacio Valley Road about a half mile west.

The trail takes you past downtown Alamo and winds through a residential greenbelt until it reaches Danville's charming downtown area. You'll find parking, restrooms, drinking fountains, and lots of dining and shopping options. Rail history buffs will want to check out the restored Southern Pacific Depot, circa 1891, which is listed on the National Register of Historic Places and houses the Museum of the San Ramon Valley.

South of Danville the trail passes Bishop Ranch business park, a major employment hub, and continues through San Ramon. Stay alert for golf cart crossings as you cut through the golf course and continue south to the Dublin BART station. Look for ground stencils to guide you through the station, the parking lot, and back onto the trail.

At Stoneridge Drive in Pleasanton, the trail crosses the Arroyo Mocho Trail (see page 15). To stay on the Iron Horse, follow the signs (most are pavement decals) heading southeast another 2 miles to Stanley Boulevard, where the trail then veers east toward Livermore. Enjoy beautiful views of the adjacent Shadow Cliffs Regional Recreation Area. The current trail terminus is at Isabel Avenue, but plans are in the works to extend it farther east to downtown Livermore.

When fully completed, the trail will span 55 miles and connect Suisun Bay and Martinez in the north to Pleasanton in the south and downtown Livermore to the east.

CONTACT ebparks.org/trails/interpark/iron-horse

PARKING

Parking areas are listed from north to south. Select parking areas for the trail are listed below. For a detailed list of parking areas and other waypoints, go to **TrailLink.com™**. *Indicates that at least one accessible parking space is available.*

CONCORD* Iron Horse Parking Lot on Lisa Lane, 0.2 mile east of Monument Blvd. (37.9454, -122.0513).

WALNUT CREEK* Pleasant Hill BART station, 1365 Treat Blvd. (37.9289, -122.0568); parking fees may apply (visit **bart.gov/guide/parking** for more information).

WALNUT CREEK* Walnut Creek BART station, 200 Ygnacio Valley Road (37.9058, -122.0668); parking fees may apply (visit **bart.gov/guide/parking** for more information).

ALAMO* Danville Blvd. at Rudgear Road (37.8791, -122.0503).

DANVILLE* Museum of the San Ramon Valley, 205 Railroad Ave. (37.8205, -122.0003).

SAN RAMON* 3410 Fostoria Way (37.7830, -121.9687).

SAN RAMON Central Park, 12501 Alcosta Blvd. (37.7654, -121.9536).

DUBLIN* Don Biddle Community Park, 6100 Horizon Pkwy. (37.7069, -121.9029).

PLEASANTON* Creekside Park, 5601 W. Las Positas Blvd. (37.6909, -121.8835).

PLEASANTON BMX Park, 3320 Stanley Blvd. (37.6705, -121.85351).

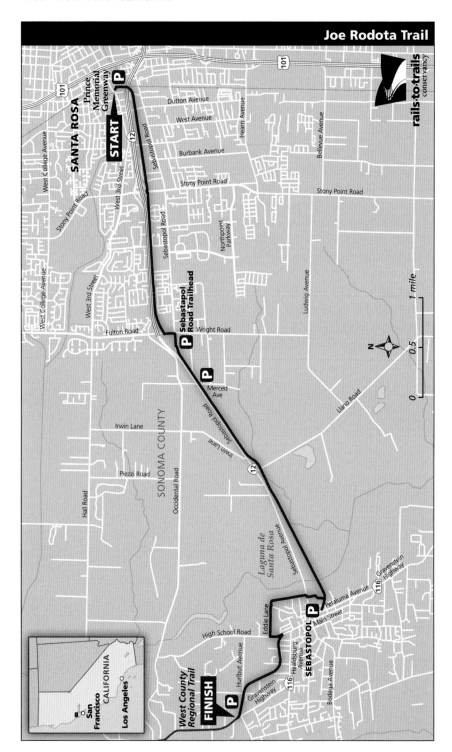

Joe Rodota Trail

Named for the first director of Sonoma County Regional Parks, the Joe Rodota Trail offers some of the county's most sweeping rural vistas. The rail-trail is built along the corridor of the old Petaluma and Santa Rosa Railway, which once ran between Santa Rosa, Petaluma, and Sebastopol. Seamlessly linked with the West County Regional Trail (see page 251), the rail-trail is part of a developing 2,600-miles-plus Bay Area regional trail network being spearheaded by the Bay Area Trails Collaborative (**railsto trails.org/bay-area**) and Rails-to-Trails Conservancy as a TrailNation™ project to increase safe walking, biking, and trail access for millions of Bay Area residents.

In Santa Rosa, the trail begins at a pedestrian/bicycle bridge intersection with the Prince Memorial Greenway. However, the recommended—and more scenic—route begins 3.1 miles farther west at the Sebastopol Road Trailhead along CA 12 (just west of N. Wright Road). Although this segment heads southwest paralleling the highway, a wide, brushy, and tree-filled median between trail and road provides a pleasant experience.

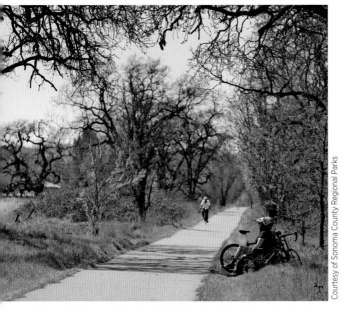

Emerging into scenic farmland, the trail evokes the area's pastoral heritage.

County
Sonoma

Endpoints
Prince Memorial Greenway, 0.2 mile southwest of W. Third St. and Railroad St. (Santa Rosa); West County Regional Trail at Mill Station Road and CA 116/Gravenstein Highway N. (Sebastopol)

Mileage
8.5

Type
Rail-Trail

Roughness Rating
1

Surface
Asphalt

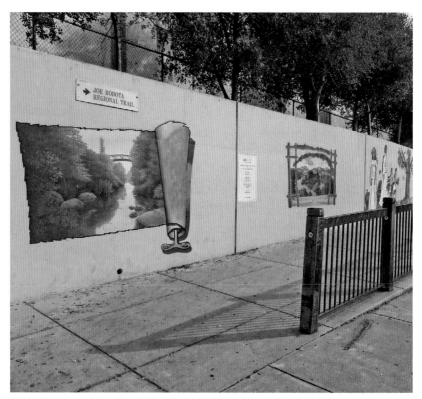

The trail passes a collaborative mural by the lead artists and apprentices of Artstart, a nonprofit arts organization.   TrailLink user tommyonbike

The trail soon emerges into scenic farmland evoking the area's pastoral heritage. The trail runs along a creek and meanders through the Laguna de Santa Rosa, the largest freshwater wetland complex in Sonoma County. If you're lucky, you may encounter a bald eagle, a white pelican, or an osprey. Note that there are unimproved trail crossings at Merced Avenue (0.4 mile from the Sebastopol Road Trailhead) and at Llano Road (1.5 miles from the trailhead), requiring caution by trail users.

Approaching Sebastopol, you'll come to a signed intersection with an accompanying trail map. Here, you can either go straight to CA 116/Petaluma Avenue, where you'll find a trailhead and parking area near charming downtown Sebastopol, or turn right, following signs for Graton and Forestville (the latter option allows you to pick up the West County Regional Trail north of town).

The Joe Rodota Trail crosses CA 12 at the signalized Morris Street intersection, then continues as an on-street connection (via bike lanes and sidewalks) heading north on Morris Street, skirting the Barlow commercial district and the eastern edge of town. About 0.4 mile from the CA 12 intersection, Morris Street curves west, and you'll soon find the signed trail on your right paralleling Eddie Lane. For part of this next segment, you'll be sharing the road right-of-way with vehicles on Eddie Lane. After passing a high school, the trail brings you to North Main Street, where you'll turn left and go 0.1 mile using bike lines until you turn right again at the signed trail. Here, the wooded path is a heavily used commuter route connecting adjacent neighborhoods to the high school and downtown Sebastopol. After about a mile, the trail feeds into CA 116/Gravenstein Highway North, where you'll see official signage marking the transition to the West County Regional Trail.

While horseback riding is permitted for the entirety of the trail, there is no equestrian parking available in the designated trail parking lots.

CONTACT parks.sonomacounty.ca.gov/visit/find-a-park/joe-rodota-trail

PARKING

Parking areas are listed from east to west. *Indicates that at least one accessible parking space is available.*

SANTA ROSA Olive Park on Hazel or Orange St. (38.4344, -122.7189); street parking only.

SANTA ROSA* Sebastopol Road Trailhead, west end of Sebastopol Road (38.4243, -122.7726).

SANTA ROSA Merced Ave. and Joe Rodota Trail (38.4207, -122.7788). Limited parking is available on the east and west side of Merced Ave. where the trail intersects the road.

SEBASTOPOL* CA 116/Petaluma Ave. Trailhead, 400 feet north of Fannen Ave. and 0.1 mile south of CA 12/Sebastopol Ave. (38.4004, -122.8222).

SEBASTOPOL Sebastopol Charter School, 1111 Gravenstein Hwy. N. (38.4133, -122.8418).

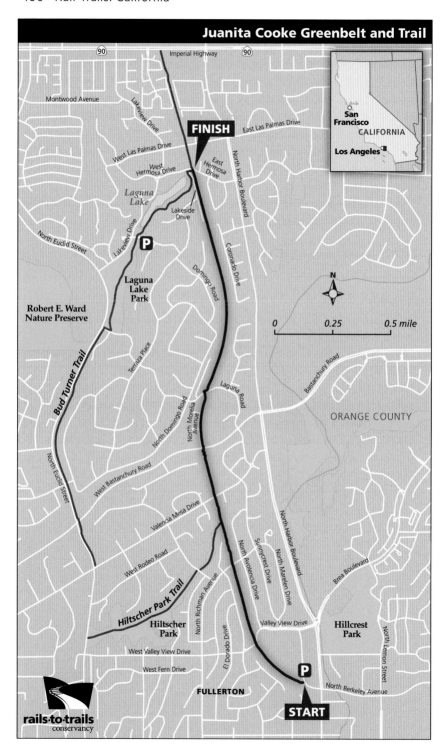

Juanita Cooke Greenbelt and Trail

The Juanita Cooke Greenbelt and Trail recalls a time when many residents of the once sleepy burg of Fullerton in Orange County enjoyed horseback riding for sport and recreation. Equestrians are still welcome—as are walkers and bicyclists—on this 2.5-mile soft-surface path named for the woman who was instrumental in converting this corridor from rail to trail.

The mostly packed-dirt trail runs from the vicinity of downtown Fullerton north into the suburbs. The scents of flowering shrubs and citrus trees sweeten the air in the neighborhoods. Along the southern section, the owners of the adjacent homes have beautified both sides of the trail with lush gardens and tall palms.

The trail follows the local route of the Pacific Electric Railway, which launched in 1901 and spread across 1,100 miles of track throughout Southern California. Known for its Red Cars, the railway arrived in Fullerton in 1917 to carry passengers and haul the lucrative citrus crop to market. Modern highways and the proliferation of cars and trucks doomed the interurban electric railway by the late 1940s.

County
Orange

Endpoints
N. Berkeley Ave., 400 feet west of N. Harbor Blvd. (Fullerton); W. Hermosa Dr. and Lakeside Dr. (Fullerton)

Mileage
2.5

Type
Rail-Trail

Roughness Rating
2

Surface
Dirt

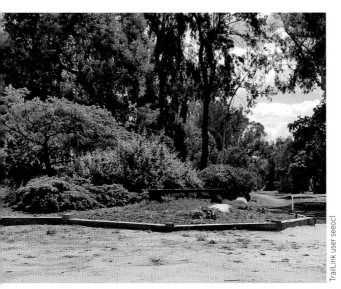

TrailLink user seeocl

This soft-surface path is named for the woman who was instrumental in its rail-trail conversion.

Meanwhile, sprawling development was overtaking areas where equestrians could enjoy their pastime. In the early 1960s, members of the Fullerton Recreational Riders, with the help of city commissioner Juanita Cooke, acquired permission from the city to improve the defunct railbed as a bridle trail. As time passed, the city got involved in improving the trail for all users.

The southern trailhead at the courthouse complex on North Berkeley Avenue is a good place to start your explorations. This is also the start of the Fullerton Loop, a mountain biking trail that incorporates several trails and streets for a dozen miles.

The Juanita Cooke Greenbelt and Trail rolls through a corridor flanked by trees and backyard fences. In less than a mile, you'll pass the Hiltscher Park Trail, which runs alongside a creek in a narrow park for 1 mile. In another 0.3 mile, switchbacks lead downhill to Bastanchury Road. To reach the continuation of the trail, cross the street, take a sidewalk along North Morelia Avenue for 0.2 mile, and then cross Laguna Road.

The greenbelt continues among residences to a 1917 bridge crossing over disused Union Pacific Railroad tracks. Nearly a mile past Laguna Road, the greenbelt meets the Bud Turner Trail (also named for a local trail advocate) on the left. The 2-mile Turner Trail passes tranquil Laguna Lake on its way to a park and equestrian center that has riding rings, show rings, and a grandstand and is home to the Fullerton Recreation Riders.

Although the greenbelt officially ends at West Hermosa Drive, a rough informal path continues north for a half mile to CA 90/Imperial Highway.

CONTACT cityoffullerton.com/government/departments/parks-recreation

---

PARKING

Parking areas are located within Fullerton and are listed from south to north. *Indicates that at least one accessible parking space is available.*

FULLERTON COURTHOUSE* 1231 N. Berkeley Ave., 0.1 mile northwest of N. Harbor Blvd. (33.8801, -117.9264).

LAGUNA LAKE PARK* 886 Clarion Dr. (33.9062, -117.9382); this parking lot is located on the Bud Turner Trail, 0.4 mile southwest of its connection with the Juanita Cooke Trail.

The Lafayette-Moraga Regional Trail in San Francisco's East Bay suburbs may be unique, as it began as a mule train. Mule trains originally plodded along the corridor from the Berkeley Hills through now populous Moraga Valley to haul redwoods to Sacramento.

The popular 7.7-mile trail (it's fairly busy on weekends) runs slightly upgrade from Lafayette to Moraga. While much of the trail passes through bedroom communities, long stretches are nestled in greenbelts with eye-catching views of nearby ridges whose colors shift from emerald in the wet winters to buff in the dry summers.

The trail is also part of a developing 2,600-miles-plus Bay Area regional trail network being spearheaded by the Bay Area Trails Collaborative (**railstotrails.org/bay-area**) and Rails-to-Trails Conservancy as a TrailNation™ project to increase safe walking, biking, and trail access for millions of Bay Area residents.

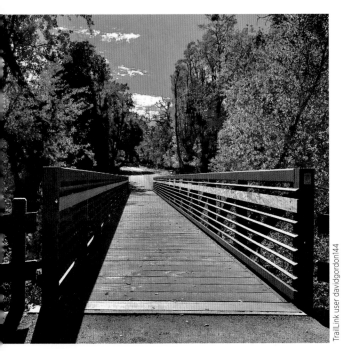

TrailLink user davidgordon144

Following Las Trampas and Moraga Creeks, the trail crosses over both a handful of times.

County
Contra Costa

Endpoints
Olympic Blvd. Staging Area at Olympic Blvd. near Pleasant Hill Road (Lafayette); Valle Vista Staging Area on Canyon Road, 0.6 mile east of Pinehurst Road (Moraga)

Mileage
7.7

Type
Rail-Trail

Roughness Rating
1

Surface
Asphalt, Concrete

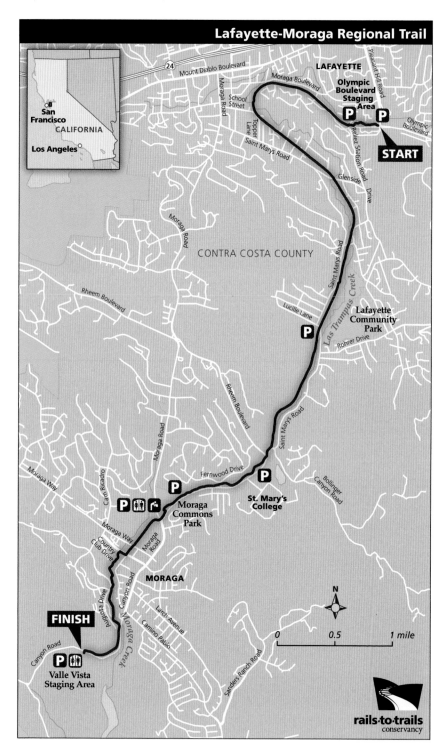

Lafayette-Moraga Regional Trail

After the 19th-century mule trains disappeared, they were replaced by railroads running steam locomotives until the Oakland, Antioch & Eastern Railway launched an electric interurban rail line in 1913. Becoming the Sacramento Northern Railway in 1920, the railroad hauled passengers and freight between San Francisco/Oakland and Chico. The interurban service ended in 1941.

The corridor remained vacant until local residents Lynn Hiden and Avon Wilson sought an alternative route to their children's schools. These self-described "PTA ladies who were able to persist" involved the cities of Lafayette and Moraga, as well as the East Bay Regional Park District, in the creation of a trail. The first segment opened in 1976 as one of the nation's earliest rail-trails.

Today, bicyclists, walkers, and equestrians share the trail, which starts in Lafayette at the corner of Pleasant Hill Road and Olympic Boulevard and runs mostly southwest along St. Marys Road to the Valle Vista staging area on Canyon Road in Moraga. It's also used by commuters, as it comes within a mile of the Lafayette BART station.

From the starting point, the trail makes a half loop to the northwest to avoid a finger of Las Trampas Ridge. As is common along most of the route, the trail then passes through a partly shady corridor flanked by suburban homes.

After about 3.5 miles, the trail passes picnic grounds and athletic fields at the 68-acre Lafayette Community Park, which is nestled between St. Marys Road and Las Trampas Creek. Remnants of pear and walnut orchards remain along the creek, where tree frogs and newts make their homes. You might catch a quick game of bocce ball being played here.

Leaving Lafayette, the trail goes through areas of open grassland and oak woodland for about 1.5 miles until it arrives at the St. Mary's College campus on the outskirts of Moraga. A mile farther is the 40-acre Moraga Commons Park, where there's a skate park and other amenities, including a water spray feature. After passing through a commercial district, the trail leaves the city center behind as it continues along Moraga Creek.

A landslide in southern Moraga in 2017 has disconnected the final half mile of trail to the Valle Vista Staging Area. To reach the trailhead, hop onto Canyon Road and head southwest 0.5 mile. Repairs have been underway; check the trail website below for updates. To access the hiking trails emanating from Valle Vista, contact the East Bay Regional Municipal Utility District (**ebmud.com /recreation**) for a hiking permit.

Closure Notice: Due to the 2022–2023 storms, a half-mile section of the Lafayette-Moraga Regional Trail from Valle Vista to Westchester Street is closed until further notice. Visit the website below for details.

CONTACT ebparks.org/trails/interpark/lafayette-moraga

continued on next page

PARKING

Parking areas are listed from north to south. *Indicates that at least one accessible parking space is available.*

LAFAYETTE* Olympic Boulevard Staging Area, Olympic Blvd. near Pleasant Hill Road (37.8860, -122.0943).

LAFAYETTE* Olympic Boulevard Staging Area, Reliez Station Road and Olympic Blvd. (37.8862, -122.0975).

LAFAYETTE Lucille Lane Staging Area, St. Marys Road and S. Lucille Lane (37.8616, -122.1018).

MORAGA* St. Marys Road Staging Area, 1913 St. Marys Road, between St. Marys Pkwy. and Rheem Blvd. (37.8450, -122.1106).

MORAGA* St. Marys Road, 0.3 mile east of Moraga Road (7.8403, -122.1244).

MORAGA* St. Marys Road, 0.1 mile east of Moraga Road (37.8394, -122.1257).

MORAGA* Valle Vista Staging Area, Canyon Road, 0.6 mile east of Pinehurst Road (37.8224, -122.1377).

The Lake Almanor Recreation Trail is much hillier than the simple, flat shoreline hike its name might suggest. The lake is a hydroelectric project that dates back more than 100 years to 1914 and is operated by the Pacific Gas & Electric Co.

This 11-mile trail through pleasant surroundings in the Lassen National Forest features a paved surface that is rutted and collects plenty of fallen forest debris, including the occasional tree. A hybrid or mountain bike is recommended instead of a road bike, and users of many types of wheelchairs could encounter problems. In-line skating is not recommended due to the conditions. It is also recommended that trail users review the state's wildfire restrictions before hitting the trail: **rtc.li/blm-fire-info.**

The area around Lake Almanor was touched by the 2021 Dixie Fire that swept across five northern California

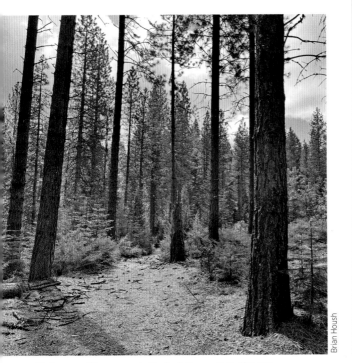

Trail users will be surrounded by the tall evergreens of Lassen National Forest.

County
Plumas

Endpoints
Humbug Humboldt Cross Road/FR 27N52, 0.1 mile east of CA 89/Volcanic Legacy Scenic Byway (Canyondam); Canyon Dam Boat Launch and Day Use Area, end of FR 27N02, 0.4 mile east of CA 89 (Canyondam)

Mileage
11

Type
Greenway/Non-Rail-Trail

Roughness Rating
2

Surface
Asphalt

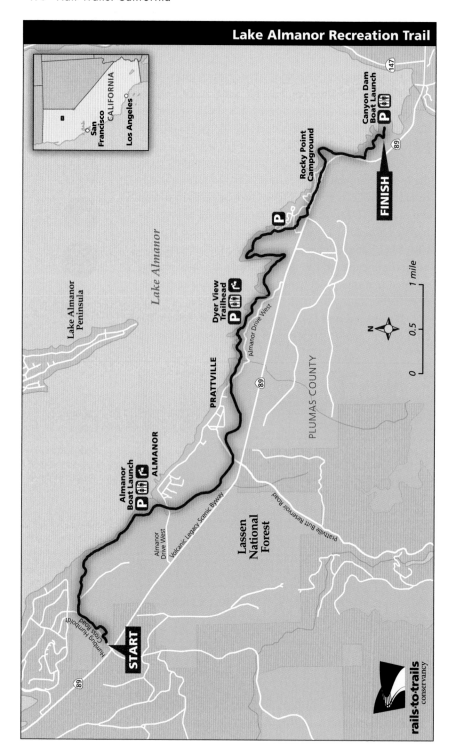

counties, but it was spared significant damage. Wildflowers were reported growing in the burn areas during the spring after the fire.

The northwestern end point doesn't have a parking lot—just an unpaved clearing in the woods where a vehicle could drop someone off. Parking is available 2.3 miles down the trail at the Almanor Boat Launch, which is accessible from Almanor Drive West.

The northwestern half of the trail is almost entirely wooded. Starting at the clearing on Forest Road 27N52/Humbug Humboldt Cross Road, the trail heads toward the lake and then alongside it to a boat launch. From there, it meanders away from the lake as it passes near the communities of Almanor and Prattville, both of which have a restaurant open in season. While lake views are relatively few, trail users will appreciate the serenity of the expansive conifer forest. Undulating hills and occasional obstacles provide fun for users seeking an experience loosely reminiscent of mountain biking.

The trail boasts more lake vistas about 5.5 miles from the start, including Mount Lassen Volcano in Lassen Volcanic National Park to the northwest. In 1915, Lassen Peak erupted, sending fiery ash 7 miles into the air and a gray ash cloud as far as Nevada. Until the eruption of Mount St. Helens in 1980, it was the most recent active volcano in the Cascade Range. The Cascade Volcanoes are a part of a volcanic chain known as the Ring of Fire—hot spots along the edges of plates under the Pacific Ocean bordering the Americas, Asia, and Oceania. Lassen Peak is the world's largest plug-dome volcano.

In 3 miles, the trail passes the Rocky Point Campground with a picnic area and a sandy beach. The trail ends about 2 miles farther south at the Canyon Dam Boat Launch. The lake spillway into the North Fork Feather River is 0.7 mile south on CA 89/Volcano Legacy Scenic Byway.

CONTACT rtc.li/lake-almanor-rec-trail

PARKING

Parking areas are listed from northwest to southeast. *Indicates that at least one accessible parking space is available.*

ALMANOR* Almanor Boat Launch (north of Prattville), Almanor Dr. W., 1.1 miles east of its northern intersection with CA 89 (40.2211, -121.1782).

PRATTVILLE Dyer View Trailhead, Almanor Dr. W., 0.6 mile northeast of its southern intersection with CA 89 (40.2023, -121.1366).

CANYONDAM Rocky Point Campground, Rocky Point Campground Road, 0.1 mile north of CA 89 (40.1951, -121.1159).

CANYONDAM* Canyon Dam Boat Ramp and Day Use Area, end of FR 27N02, 0.4 mile east of CA 89 (40.1790, -121.0942).

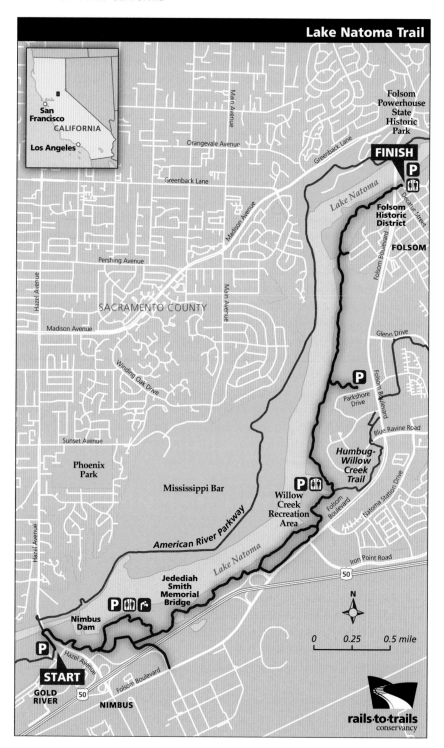

Lake Natoma Trail

San Francisco
CALIFORNIA
Los Angeles

Folsom Powerhouse State Historic Park

FINISH

Folsom Historic District

FOLSOM

Lake Natoma

Orangevale Avenue

Greenback Lane

Greenback Lane

Main Avenue

Madison Avenue

Decatur Street

Folsom Boulevard

Pershing Avenue

Hazel Avenue

SACRAMENTO COUNTY

Madison Avenue

Main Avenue

Glenn Drive

Folsom Boulevard

Parkshore Drive

Winding Oak Drive

Blue Ravine Road

Sunset Avenue

Humbug-Willow Creek Trail

Phoenix Park

Mississippi Bar

Willow Creek Recreation Area

Folsom Boulevard

Natoma Station Drive

American River Parkway

Iron Point Road

50

Lake Natoma

Hazel Avenue

Jedediah Smith Memorial Bridge

N

Nimbus Dam

0   0.25   0.5 mile

START

GOLD RIVER   50

Hazel Avenue

Folsom Boulevard

NIMBUS

rails·to·trails
conservancy

Many consider the Lake Natoma Trail to be a part of the American River Parkway (see page 13), but it is a distinct trail that connects with the parkway as part of a larger trail system in Folsom. The trail spans 5.5 miles of mostly flat, paved terrain that closely hugs Lake Natoma between Nimbus Dam and the Folsom Historic District, offering visitors the chance to take a scenic journey with many benches and picnic tables along the way for stopping to enjoy the views. The route is partially shaded by trees, and as trail users make their way from south to north, they will pass vast grassy plains to the right and have magnificent waterside views of Lake Natoma to the left.

At its southern end, the Lake Natoma Trail intersects with the American River Parkway near the Nimbus Fish Ladder. The trailhead here has a parking area overlooking the Nimbus Dam, where the American River meets Lake Natoma, and is a short distance from Nimbus Flat State Recreation Area, a small park with a lakefront beach and a boat ramp.

County
Sacramento

Endpoints
American River Parkway, 500 feet north of Gold Country Blvd. and Nimbus Road (Gold River); Gold Lake Dr., 0.1 mile north of Leidesdorff St. (Folsom)

Mileage
5.5

Type
Greenway/Non-Rail-Trail

Roughness Rating
1

Surface
Asphalt

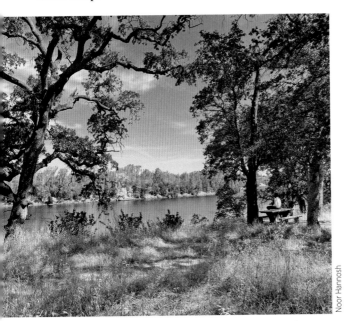

Noor Hannosh

Winding through lakefront recreation areas, the trail provides outdoor access in the Sacramento suburb of Folsom.

The only surface change of the route occurs 1.4 miles into your journey when you reach a wooden bridge that is somewhat bumpy. In another 1.4 miles, you will arrive at the Willow Creek Recreation Area, where there are wheelchair-accessible restrooms, a parking area, picnic tables, beach access to the lake, and a boat ramp. In 0.1 mile, the Lake Natoma Trail intersects with the Humbug–Willow Creek Trail (see page 91), then continues 2.4 miles to trail's end and downtown Folsom's historic district.

In the Folsom Historic District, visitors will find shops, restaurants, museums, an amphitheater, and a light-rail station. If you want to keep the adventure going, the Folsom Powerhouse State Historic Park, Folsom Parkway Rail Trail, and Johnny Cash Trail are only a short distance away.

CONTACT rtc.li/california-parks

PARKING

Parking areas are listed from south to north. Select parking areas for the trail are listed below. For a detailed list of parking areas and other waypoints, go to **TrailLink.com**™. *Indicates that at least one accessible parking space is available.*

GOLD RIVER American River Fishing Access, Gold Country Blvd. and Nimbus Road (38.6322, -121.2243).

RANCHO CORDOVA* 1901 Hazel Ave. (38.6342, -121.2205).

RANCHO CORDOVA* Nimbus Flat State Recreation Area, 0.1 mile east of Hazel Ave. (38.6347, -121.2167).

FOLSOM* Willow Creek Recreation Area; the entrance to the parking lot is on Folsom Blvd., 400 feet east of Natoma Station Dr. (38.6488, -121.1904).

FOLSOM* Parkshore Trailhead, Parkshore Dr., 0.1 mile west of Folsom Blvd. (38.6590, -121.1851).

FOLSOM* Folsom Historic District, 905 Leidesdorff St. (38.6770, -121.1785).

The name *Lands End Trail* isn't an exaggeration. This San Francisco trail skirts the edge of North America on rocky cliffs overlooking the Pacific Ocean. The 1.6-mile trail offers spectacular views of the Golden Gate Bridge and old shipwrecks, as well as a full complement of marine mammals and seabirds.

The path meanders through the Golden Gate National Recreation Area, where you can also find the Legion of Honor art museum and the now-closed swank Cliff House restaurant, as well as ruins of a beach resort and public baths. The Lands End Trail is a segment of the developing California Coastal Trail—a network of bicycling and hiking trails that, when complete, will stretch along the coastline for 1,230 miles from Oregon to the Mexican border—and is also part of a developing 2,600-miles-plus Bay Area regional trail network being spearheaded by the Bay Area Trails Collaborative (**railstotrails.org/bay-area**)

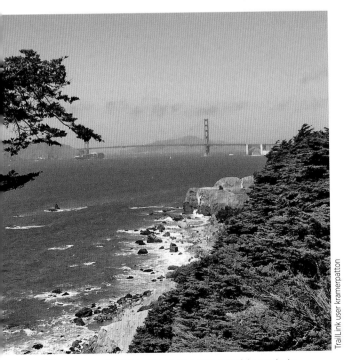

TrailLink user kramerpatton

Visitors can see the Golden Gate Bridge from one of the overlooks.

County
San Francisco

Endpoints
Merrie Way and Point Lobos Ave. (San Francisco); El Camino del Mar, just west of 32nd Ave. (San Francisco)

Mileage
1.6

Type
Rail-Trail

Roughness Rating
2

Surface
Crushed Stone, Dirt

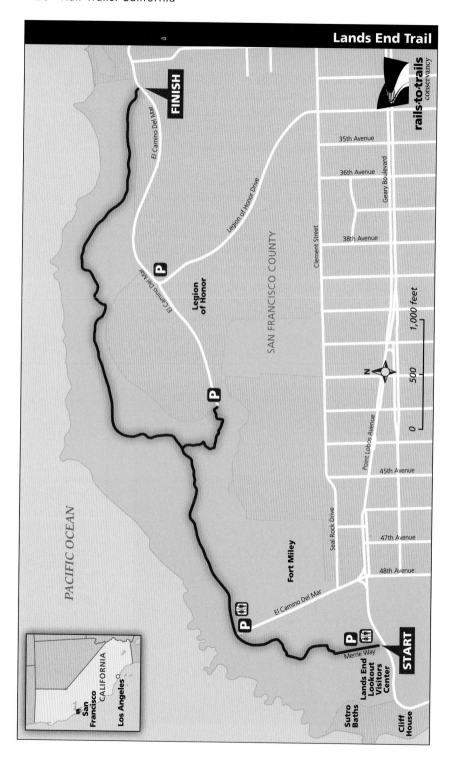

Lands End Trail

FINISH

rails-to-trails
conservancy

35th Avenue

36th Avenue

38th Avenue

Clement Street

Geary Boulevard

El Camino Del Mar

Legion of Honor Drive

P

Legion
of Honor

SAN FRANCISCO COUNTY

El Camino Del Mar

1,000 feet

N

500

0

P

Point Lobos Avenue

45th Avenue

Seal Rock Drive

47th Avenue

Fort Miley

48th Avenue

PACIFIC OCEAN

El Camino Del Mar

P

P

Merrie Way

START

Lands End
Lookout
Visitors
Center

Sutro
Baths

Cliff
House

CALIFORNIA

San
Francisco

Los Angeles

and Rails-to-Trails Conservancy as a TrailNation™ project to increase safe walking, biking, and trail access for millions of Bay Area residents.

The Lands End Trail, one of several in the park, follows the route of the Park and Cliff House Railway, which carried passengers by steam train and later electric trolley to oceanside tourist destinations beginning in 1888. A landslide wiped out a section of track in 1925, ending rail service.

A convenient starting point is the parking lot at Merrie Way, named after the Sutro Pleasure Grounds at Merrie Way, an amusement park that operated there from 1896 to 1900. The lot now features the Lands End Lookout Visitor Center. Before heading onto the Lands End Trail at the north end of the lot, you might want to take the steps downhill on the left to explore the historic Sutro Baths ruins, where, from 1896 to 1966, visitors soaked in heated seawater and enjoyed shows and sports. A quarter mile west on Point Lobos Avenue is the aptly named Cliff House, a historic restaurant that closed in 2020.

Heading north onto the Lands End Trail, you'll pass through groves of cypress and eucalyptus to views of the coast and the rocky shores that have claimed more than a few unlucky ships. At low tide in clear weather, you might see parts of old ships sticking out of the sand. If the pea-soup fog has rolled in, you won't see the wrecks, but you'll understand why so many ships crashed onto this shoreline.

The overlooks here also feature breathtaking views—weather permitting—of the Golden Gate Bridge and the Marin Headlands across the mouth of the bay, with the best views at sunset. Be sure to stay on the trails, as the cliff faces are treacherous.

About 0.6 mile along the trail, a right fork heads 0.3 mile uphill to the Legion of Honor art museum, which houses several art collections. Built in Beaux Arts style in 1921, the palatial building commands a view of the San Francisco skyline.

Back on the trail—referred to as Coastal Trail in places—the crushed-stone path becomes dirt after the fork. You'll then come upon some stairs, where bikes are prohibited.

The trail ends at El Camino Del Mar, which you can take back (west) for a loop outing. Along the way, you'll pass the remains of Fort Miley, part of the coastal defenses launched in the late 1890s.

CONTACT nps.gov/goga

continued on next page

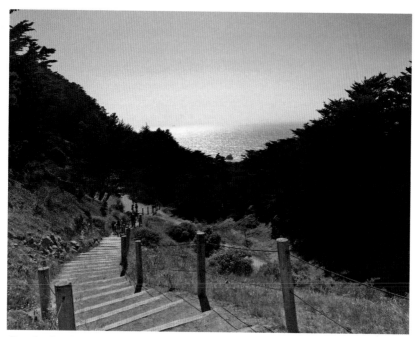

Steps heading down from the trail lead to additional attractions along the shoreline.
TrailLink user kramerpatton

PARKING

Parking areas are located within San Francisco and are listed from west to east. *Indicates that at least one accessible parking space is available.*

MERRIE WAY PARKING* Point Lobos Ave., just west of El Camino Del Mar (37.7801, -122.5104).

EL CAMINO DEL MAR PARKING* El Camino Del Mar, 0.2 mile northwest of Point Lobos Ave. (37.7824, -122.5110).

LEGION OF HONOR PARKING* El Camino Del Mar and Legion of Honor Dr. (37.7855, -122.4995).

On-street parking is provided along El Camino Del Mar at Seal Rock Dr. (37.7808, -122.5101).

The Los Gatos Creek Trail runs for nearly 11 miles along Los Gatos Creek from San Jose to Los Gatos. It is part of a developing 2,600-miles-plus Bay Area regional trail network being spearheaded by the Bay Area Trails Collaborative (**railstotrails.org/bay-area**) and Rails-to-Trails Conservancy as a TrailNation™ project to increase safe walking, biking, and trail access for millions of Bay Area residents. While the northern Dupont Street endpoint has no parking or facilities (just a handful of street parking spaces are available), the Del Monte Dog Park is 0.2 mile down the trail and offers restrooms, water, picnic areas, and on-street parking.

Less than a mile along the paved trail, there is a 1.4-mile gap in the trail that can be bridged with an on-street connection through San Jose. This route begins at Lonus Street. Take your first left (after 0.1 mile) onto Lincoln Avenue. After 0.2 mile, take a right onto Glen Eyrie Avenue, then another right onto Willow Street in 0.7 mile.

County
Santa Clara

Endpoints
Dupont St., south of W. San Carlos St. (San Jose); dead end of Lonus St., 0.1 mile east of Lincoln St. (San Jose); Meridian Ave., 0.2 mile north of Westwood Dr. (San Jose); Alma Bridge Road, 0.5 mile northeast of Santa Cruz Hwy. in Lexington Reservoir County Park (Los Gatos)

Mileage
10.7

Type
Greenway/Non-Rail-Trail

Roughness Rating
1

Surface
Asphalt, Concrete, Gravel

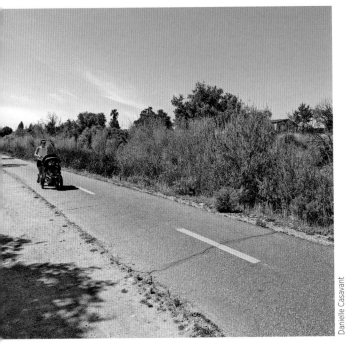

Danielle Casavant

Winding through residential neighborhoods along its namesake creek, the trail connects San José and Los Gatos.

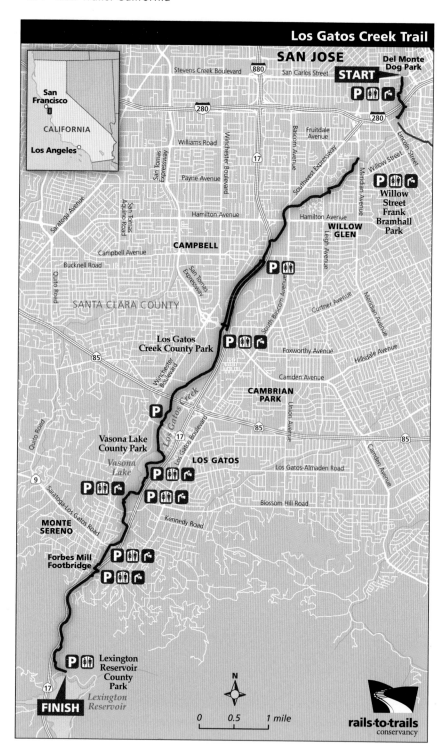

Los Gatos Creek Trail

(At the intersection of Willow Street and Glen Eyrie Avenue, the Willow Street Frank Bramhall Park offers a parking lot, restrooms, water, and picnic sites.) In 0.2 mile, turn right on Meridian Avenue; in 0.2 mile, the trail picks up again, headed southwest, north of Westwood Drive.

Once you rejoin the trail, it winds through residential neighborhoods, behind apartment complexes, businesses, and nearby schools. Much of the trail is surrounded by abundant greenery. There are several neighborhood access points along this new section of trail, making it a great way for area residents to take nonmotorized routes to school and other community spots. About 2.2 miles down this section of trail, just past the helpfully marked Campbell Avenue underpass, the trail splits with a bridge over Los Gatos Creek, giving you the choice of riding along the east or west banks of the creek. At 3.3 miles, make sure to take the last bridge crossing to the right (northwest) side of the trail if you aren't already there, as the left (southeast) side ends shortly thereafter.

At mile 3.6 is Los Gatos Creek County Park; it offers parking for a fee, as well as restrooms and picnic areas. This is a very popular place to access the trail and is about halfway between the two endpoints. With multiple ponds, the park is a great spot for birding and observing wildlife.

South of Los Gatos Creek County Park, you'll reach a free trailside parking lot in 1.5 miles, located at Charter Oaks Drive in Los Gatos. The trail continues another 2 miles before meeting up with Vasona Lake County Park. This full-service park offers numerous fee-based parking lots, public restrooms, and water. The trail winds through the park and alongside a reservoir with shady spots for a picnic. The park and trail in this area are heavily used by bikers, walkers, and joggers and are family friendly.

The next 1.5 miles of trail meanders through a parklike setting to the Forbes Mill Footbridge spanning CA 17. After the overpass, the trail changes to packed gravel suitable for walking, jogging, and most bikes but not advised for wheelchair use. This section of trail is wooded and feels far more rural than previous sections. The last 0.5 mile to the endpoint at the Lexington Reservoir County Park requires a steep uphill climb on loose gravel. The 950-acre park (including the reservoir) is an oasis of nature in an urban area. It has fee-based parking and offers restrooms; a public boat launch for nonmotorized boats; and quiet water recreation, including kayaks, canoes, stand-up paddleboards, and inner tubes.

CONTACT rtc.li/city-san-jose and **losgatosca.gov/907/los-gatos-creek-trail**

continued on next page

PARKING

Parking areas are listed from north to south. Select parking areas for the trail are listed below. For a detailed list of parking areas and other waypoints, go to **TrailLink.com**™. *Indicates that at least one accessible parking space is available.*

CAMPBELL* Campbell Park, Gilman Ave. and E. Campbell Ave. (37.2861, -121.9398).

CAMPBELL* Los Gatos Creek County Park, 1250 Dell Ave. (37.2698, -121.9504).

LOS GATOS Charter Oaks Dr. and Willow Hill Ct. (37.2549, -121.9625).

LOS GATOS* Vasona Lake County Park, Blossom Hill Road, 0.3 mile west of Roberts Road E. (37.2355, -121.9731).

LOS GATOS* 57 Miles Ave. (37.2243, -121.9788).

LOS GATOS Forbes Mill Footbridge, adjacent to the Forbes Mill Museum at 75 Church St. (37.2221, -121.9799).

LOS GATOS Lexington Reservoir County Park, 17770 Alma Bridge Road (37.2002, -121.9867).

On-street parking is available along W. Home St. at San Jose's Del Monte Dog Park (37.3201, -121.9050).

The scenic MacKerricher Haul Road Trail is part of an old road used to transport lumber from the Ten Mile River watershed to a mill in Fort Bragg. It hugs the Pacific coastline, traveling across a unique and environmentally sensitive sand dune area from the Pudding Creek Trestle near downtown Fort Bragg to a bit north of Ward Avenue, north of Cleone. The trail once continued to the Ten Mile River (so named because it's located 10 miles north of the Noyo River), but erosion closed this stretch in 2014. Today the trail is part of the developing California Coastal Trail—a network of bicycling and hiking trails that, when complete, will stretch along the coastline for 1,230 miles from Oregon to the Mexican border. Horseback riding is permitted for the full length of the trail, as well as from Ward Avenue to the Ten Mile River along the beach (stay in single file on the wet sand).

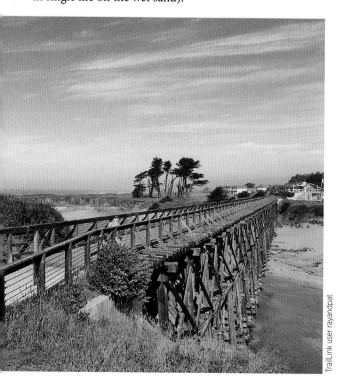

The southern end of the trail crosses over sand dunes on the Pudding Creek Trestle.

County
Mendocino

Endpoints
Dead end of Glass Beach Dr., 0.4 mile north of W. Elm St. (Fort Bragg); 0.2 mile north of the Ten Mile Beach parking lot accessible from Ward Ave. (Cleone)

Mileage
3.8

Type
Rail-Trail

Roughness Rating
2

Surface
Asphalt

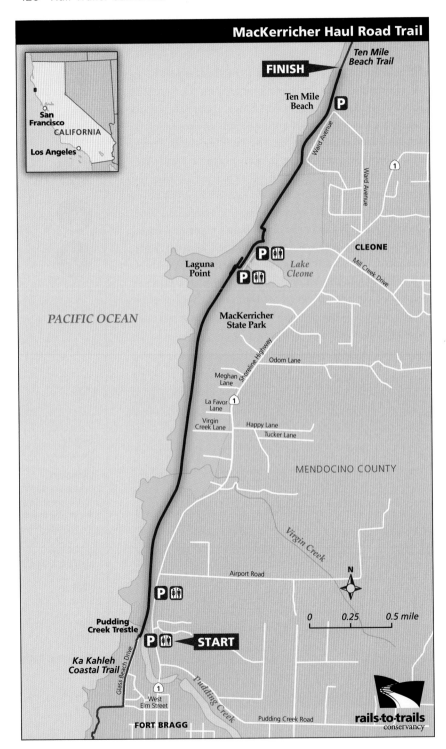

MacKerricher Haul Road Trail

FINISH

Ten Mile
Beach Trail

Ten Mile
Beach

P

San
Francisco

CALIFORNIA

Los Angeles

CLEONE

Laguna
Point

P

P

Lake
Cleone

Mill Creek Drive

Ward Avenue

Ward Avenue

1

PACIFIC OCEAN

MacKerricher
State Park

Shoreline Highway

Odom Lane

Meghan
Lane

La Favor
Lane   1

Virgin
Creek Lane   Happy Lane

Tucker Lane

MENDOCINO COUNTY

Virgin Creek

N

Airport Road

0   0.25   0.5 mile

Pudding
Creek Trestle

P

P   START

Ka Kahleh
Coastal Trail

Glass Beach Drive

Pudding Creek

1

West
Elm Street

Pudding Creek Road

FORT BRAGG

rails·to·trails
conservancy

From Pudding Creek on the south end, you cross a bridge that was the start of a lumber trading route that terminated more than 100 miles away in Eureka 150 years ago. Built in 1915–1916 by the Union Lumber Company, this bridge is the only original railroad trestle remaining on the corridor. Beyond the trestle are 4 miles of coastal bluffs. As you move along the trail, you have sweeping vistas of the ocean and may see a variety of plant and animal species. You might be able to spot the endangered western snowy plover, a bird that typically breeds in dune-related coastal habitats. Be sure to bring binoculars for whale- and seal-watching; this stretch is one of the largest uninterrupted whale-watching spots on the West Coast. Pacific gray whales can be seen on their migration route from December to April.

About a mile in, you'll head slightly downhill before crossing Virgin Creek, a great spot to sit and watch the waves and contemplate a coastline that was 3–5 miles farther west around 12,000 years ago. Continuing north, you reach sand—the geological terrain for which MacKerricher State Park is known. Dune grasses, some native and some invasive, prevent the dunes from shifting too much. After another 1.5 miles, the trail takes a short detour to merge with the adjacent Mill Creek Drive at Lake Cleone, where a section of trail has eroded away; a restroom is available at the western end of the parking lot. This nearby lovely tidal lagoon is filled with a variety of birds. Past Lake Cleone, the trail reemerges as the MacKerricher Haul Road Trail.

After the detour, the trail continues north along high bluffs, with breath-taking ocean views. A short distance ahead is the end of the rideable terrain. Turn around and head back, or park your bike and take a longer coastal walk to the Ten Mile River.

CONTACT rtc.li/mackerricher-sp

PARKING

Parking areas are listed from south to north. *Indicates that at least one accessible parking space is available.*

FORT BRAGG* Dead end of Glass Beach Dr., south of the Pudding Creek Trestle (39.4577, -123.8080).

FORT BRAGG* 1121 N. Main St./Shoreline Hwy., 600 feet south of Airport Road (39.4615, -123.8065).

FORT BRAGG* Laguna Point parking lot, Mill Creek Dr., 0.8 mile west of CA 1/ Shoreline Hwy. (39.4889, -123.7996); free day-use parking.

CLEONE Mill Creek Dr., 0.5 mile west of CA 1/Shoreline Hwy. (39.4906, -123.7953).

CLEONE* 25279 Ward Ave. (39.5019, -123.7867).

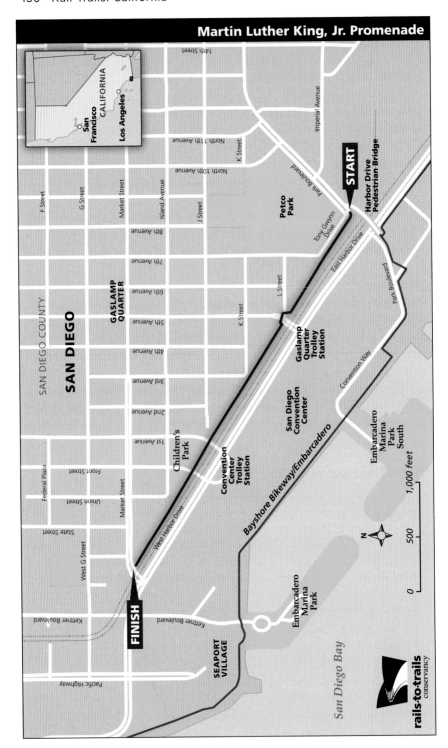

Martin Luther King, Jr. Promenade

San Diego's Martin Luther King, Jr. Promenade offers a broad, palm-lined walkway south of downtown. The 0.75-mile rail-with-trail follows the active Santa Fe Rail and San Diego Trolley tracks for its entirety, sitting adjacent to two light-rail stations (Gaslamp Quarter and Convention Center) on the Green and Silver lines for easy access to other parts of the city. Note that while bikes are prohibited on the brick pathway, the parallel Linear Park bikeway, just south of the promenade, does permit them.

At a walking pace, you can stop to appreciate the artwork and cultural touchstones along the way. Set into the grass are more than two dozen plaques engraved with the powerful and inspirational words of Dr. King. The trailside sculptures *Breaking of the Chains*, *Dream*, and *Shedding the Cloak* also commemorate the great civil rights leader.

Begin your journey at the trail's eastern end, situated between Petco Park, home to Major League Baseball's San Diego Padres, and the San Diego Convention Center. (To reach the convention center, across the railroad tracks, you can take the Harbor Drive Pedestrian Bridge, which begins

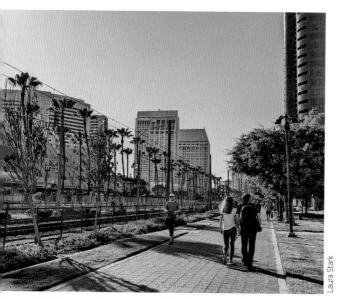

Laura Stark

Paralleling an active passenger rail line downtown, the walkway offers easy access to public transit.

County
San Diego

Endpoints
Petco Park at Tony Gwynn Dr. and Park Blvd. (San Diego); Market St. and W. Harbor Dr. (San Diego)

Mileage
0.75

Type
Rail-with-Trail

Roughness Rating
1

Surface
Brick

here.) After 0.25 mile, you'll come to your first street crossing at Fifth Avenue, where you can turn right (north) into the city's lively Gaslamp Quarter, with its trendy restaurants, bars, and hotels, or continue northwest down the promenade, which features views of skyscrapers and interesting urban architecture.

After another quarter mile, you'll reach First Avenue and the popular Children's Park, which is undergoing a major renovation to provide new amenities, including an off-leash dog park, a picnic area, exercise equipment, and restrooms.

The trail ends in the Marina District at the intersection of busy Market Street and West Harbor Drive, where you can retrace your steps to the starting point. Alternatively, from here you can follow sidewalks south down Kettner Boulevard to reach the touristy Seaport Village shopping and dining area, and the Embarcadero/Bayshore Bikeway (page 25) along the waterfront. By heading northwest along the Embarcadero, you can check out the famed USS Midway Museum, a historical naval aircraft carrier; otherwise, from Seaport Village, follow the waterfront pathway southeast back to the convention center and the start of the Martin Luther King, Jr. Promenade.

CONTACT tclf.org/martin-luther-king-jr-promenade

PARKING

While the trail does not have dedicated parking, metered parking can be found along Fifth and First Aves., which the trail crosses, or in the large paid parking lots surrounding Petco Park on the east end of the trail. The trail is also accessible via the San Diego Trolley (**sdmts .com**) from the **GASLAMP QUARTER** and **CONVENTION CENTER** stations on the Green and Silver lines.

Arguably the most iconic trail in California, the Marvin Braude Bike Trail—commonly referred to as The Strand by residents—hugs Los Angeles County's coastline from its upscale neighborhoods in the north to its historically working class (but increasingly upscale) neighborhoods in the south. While the trail travels along the beach for the majority of its 22 miles, it also takes you through a wide range of neighborhoods and landscapes. Stops at the Santa Monica Pier, the Venice Boardwalk, and the downtowns of LA's South Bay cities are a must. The trail is part of the developing California Coastal Trail—a network of bicycling and hiking trails that, when complete, will stretch along the coastline for 1,230 miles from Oregon to the Mexican border.

Begin your trip in the north at Will Rogers State Beach and the base of the Santa Monica Mountains, near the homes of many famous Hollywood actors. Take a moment to sit on a bench, watch a pickup game of beach

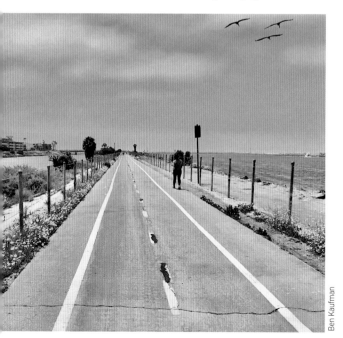

Ben Kaufman

A scenic stretch of the trail lies between Ballona Creek and the Marina del Rey inlet.

County
Los Angeles

Endpoints
Will Rogers State Beach
on Pacific Coast Hwy./
CA 1 (Los Angeles);
Via Riviera and Paseo
de la Playa (Torrance)

Mileage
22

Type
Greenway/Non-Rail-Trail

Roughness Rating
1

Surface
Asphalt, Concrete

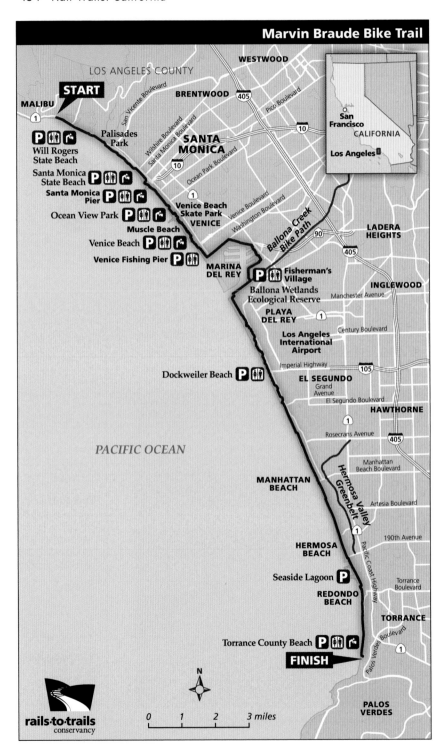

Marvin Braude Bike Trail

WESTWOOD

LOS ANGELES COUNTY

BRENTWOOD 405

START

MALIBU
1

Palisades Park

SANTA MONICA

San Vicente Boulevard
Wilshire Boulevard
Santa Monica Boulevard
Pico Boulevard

10

10

Will Rogers State Beach

Ocean Park Boulevard

Santa Monica State Beach

1

Santa Monica Pier

Venice Beach Skate Park

Venice Boulevard
Washington Boulevard

Ocean View Park

VENICE

Muscle Beach

Venice Beach

Venice Fishing Pier

MARINA DEL REY

Ballona Creek Bike Path

90

LADERA HEIGHTS

405

Fisherman's Village

INGLEWOOD

Ballona Wetlands Ecological Reserve

Manchester Avenue

PLAYA DEL REY

1

Los Angeles International Airport

Century Boulevard

Imperial Highway

105

Dockweiler Beach

EL SEGUNDO

Grand Avenue

El Segundo Boulevard

HAWTHORNE

1

Rosecrans Avenue

405

PACIFIC OCEAN

Manhattan Beach Boulevard

MANHATTAN BEACH

Hermosa Valley Greenbelt

Artesia Boulevard

1

190th Avenue

HERMOSA BEACH

Pacific Coast Highway

Seaside Lagoon

Torrance Boulevard

REDONDO BEACH

TORRANCE

Palos Verdes Boulevard

Torrance County Beach

FINISH

1

N

PALOS VERDES

rails-to-trails
conservancy

0   1   2   3 miles

San Francisco

CALIFORNIA

Los Angeles

volleyball, and breathe in the salty ocean air. As you travel south, the freeway and trail begin to diverge, with the rhythmic crashing of the Pacific Ocean's waves replacing the low hum of traffic along the Pacific Coast Highway. Cafés and cabanas crop up between the trail and the imposing cliffs, where a long row of bright-white Santa Monica hotels and condominiums are perched.

After 3.5 miles, the trail sails under the Santa Monica Pier and continues south through Santa Monica. Along the way are plentiful bathrooms, water fountains, and playgrounds, as the city takes pride in its oceanfront facilities. When you reach the Venice Boardwalk in 1.8 mile, the trail splits in two: a bicycle-only facility closer to the ocean, and a grand pedestrian promenade with a lively mix of shops, eateries, and street entertainers.

The beachfront path ends at the Venice Fishing Pier, and the route turns inland to go around Marina del Rey. At the pier, you'll turn left on Washington Boulevard for a 1-mile on-road portion. At Mildred Avenue, the paved pathway picks up again on your right. You'll take the trail for 1.4 miles until it ends at Fiji Way. Take a right on Fiji Way, following the bike lane back toward the ocean. In 0.7 mile, you'll reach a roundabout and see the entrance to the paved pathway once again. After 0.1 mile, you'll reach a T intersection overlooking Ballona Creek. Turn right to stay on the Marvin Braude Bike Trail; turning left would put you on the Ballona Creek Bike Path (see page 21). You'll follow the path along the creek until you reach the beach.

The final 12 miles of the trail through South Bay feel slightly more industrial as you travel past the Los Angeles International Airport, an oil refinery, a power plant, and a wastewater treatment facility. But don't let these land uses deter you! Nestled between them are some of the quaintest beachside communities in all of Southern California. Peel off at Manhattan Beach, Hermosa Beach, or Redondo Beach for lunch to experience a more authentic version of California beachside living. Get back on the trail for the last leg and admire the South Bay's unique architecture as it turns from extravagant single-family homes to midcentury-modern condo complexes. Enjoy a final stop in Torrance at the trail's end and see if you can spot a whale or dolphin on the horizon.

Closure Notice: Due to the 2022–2023 storms, a section of the Marvin Braude Bike Trail in Playa del Rey is damaged between the outlet of Ballona Creek and Dockweiler State Beach. A signed detour using Marine Avenue is available, and repairs are expected to be completed in summer 2023. Closure updates can be found on the Los Angeles County Public Works website: **rtc.li/pw-lacounty.**

CONTACT **beaches.lacounty.gov/la-county-beach-bike-path**

continued on next page

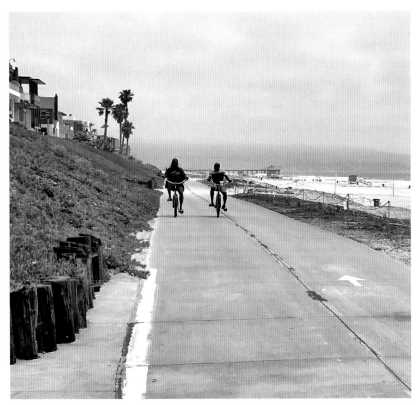

Tracing the Santa Monica Bay, the route boasts a handful of trailside beaches.   Ben Kaufman

PARKING

Parking areas are listed from north to south. Select parking areas for the trail are listed below. For a detailed list of parking areas and other waypoints, go to **TrailLink.com**™. *Indicates that at least one accessible parking space is available.*

PACIFIC PALISADES* Will Rogers State Beach, 16430 CA 1 (34.0386, -118.5426).

SANTA MONICA* Palisades Park, 772–798 CA 1/E. Pacific Coast Hwy. (34.0211, -118.5084).

SANTA MONICA* Santa Monica State Beach, 1150 E. Pacific Coast Hwy. (34.0162, -118.5019).

SANTA MONICA* Santa Monica Pier, 15 Colorado Ave. (34.0109, -118.4965).

SANTA MONICA* Ocean View Park, 2701 Barnard Way (33.9993, -118.4855).

VENICE* Venice Beach, 2100 Ocean Front Walk (33.9837, -118.4712).

VENICE* Venice Fishing Pier, 3099–3011 Ocean Front Walk (33.9790, -118.4669).

MARINA DEL REY* Fisherman's Village, 13745 Fiji Way (33.9730, -118.4459).

PLAYA DEL REY* Dockweiler Beach, Vista Del Mar and Imperial Hwy. (33.9305, -118.4356).

REDONDO BEACH* Seaside Lagoon, 161 N. Harbor Dr. (33.8449, -118.3934).

REDONDO BEACH* Torrance County Beach, 387 Paseo De La Playa (33.8126, -118.3907).

About 20 miles southwest of Yosemite National Park, the scenic Merced River Trail functions as both a bike/pedestrian trail and a lightly trafficked vehicular road used to access campsites and recreational amenities within the Merced River Recreation Area. Following the historical Yosemite Valley Railroad along the Merced River, the trail offers a relatively flat grade for intermediate skill levels. It's especially beautiful in the spring with an explosion of wildflowers that lasts from March to May.

The eastern entrance at the Briceburg Visitor Center provides parking, river access, and shade for resting or a picnic lunch along the river. Upon setting off westward from the parking lot, you will pass over a narrow bridge that accommodates both automobiles and bikes. Turn left after the bridge and follow the path west along the Merced River; going straight would take you instead to a switchbacking hiking trail up a mountainside.

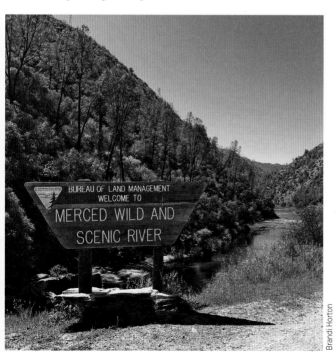

The trail offers a rugged experience within the Merced River Recreation Area west of Yosemite National Park.

Brandi Horton

County
Mariposa

Endpoints
Briceburg Visitor Center on Central Yosemite Hwy./CA 140 (Briceburg); gate located 600 feet north of Railroad Flat Campground (Midpines)

Mileage
4.9

Type
Rail-Trail

Roughness Rating
2

Surface
Gravel

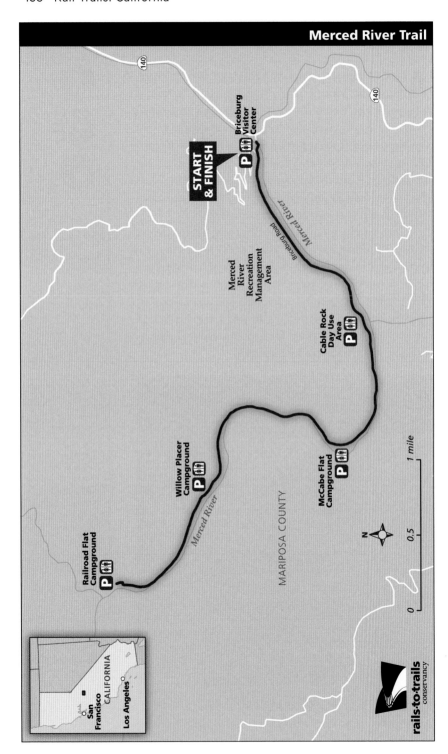

Merced River Trail

140

140

Briceburg Visitor Center

P

START & FINISH

Merced River

Briceburg Road

Merced River Recreation Management Area

Cable Rock Day Use Area

P

Willow Placer Campground

P

Merced River

MARIPOSA COUNTY

McCabe Flat Campground

P

Railroad Flat Campground

P

N

0   0.5   1 mile

CALIFORNIA

San Francisco

Los Angeles

rails-to-trails
conservancy

The Merced River will be a constant companion, and there are river access points throughout, including places to hop in for a quick swim or to go rafting. Gold prospecting and trout fishing are also common. A popular place to enjoy these activities is the Cable Rock Day Use Area, which you'll reach after 1.4 miles.

As you continue west down the gravel road maintained by the Bureau of Land Management (BLM), you may encounter the occasional vehicle sharing the road to access three campgrounds along the route, all providing restrooms and parking: McCabe Flat (1 mile west of Cable Rock), Willow Placer (1.5 miles after McCabe Flat), and Railroad Flat (0.8 mile after Willow Placer).

Although the multiuse pathway (and BLM road) ends at a gate just north of Railroad Flat Campground, adventurers can find hiking-only opportunities beyond it.

CONTACT blm.gov/visit/merced-river and mariposacounty.org/2306/merced-river-trail

PARKING

Parking areas are located within Briceburg and are listed from east to west. *Indicates that at least one accessible parking space is available.*

MERCED RIVER RECREATION MANAGEMENT AREA Central Yosemite Hwy./CA 140, 4.1 miles north of Colorado Road (37.6049, -119.9666).

CABLE ROCK DAY USE AREA Roadside parking along Briceburg Road, 1.4 miles west of Central Yosemite Hwy. (37.5943, -119.9879).

MCCABE FLAT CAMPGROUND Briceburg Road, 2.5 miles west of Central Yosemite Hwy. (37.5965, -120.0035).

WILLOW PLACER CAMPGROUND Briceburg Road, 4 miles west of Central Yosemite Hwy. (37.6103, -120.0096).

RAILROAD FLAT CAMPGROUND Briceburg Road, 4.8 miles west of Central Yosemite Hwy. (37.6172, -120.0200).

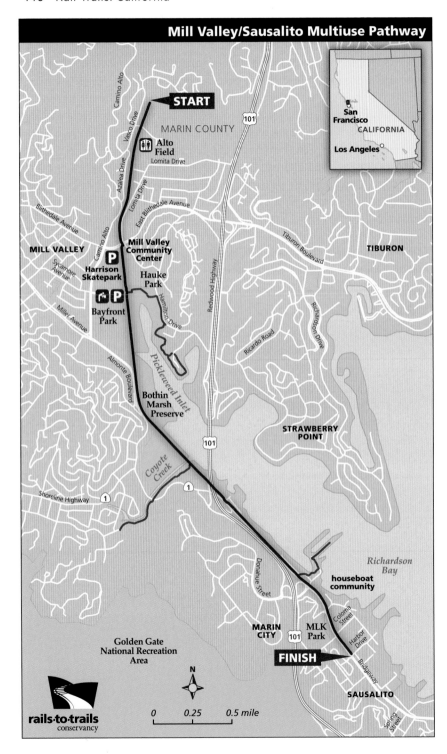

Mill Valley/Sausalito Multiuse Pathway

START

MARIN COUNTY

Alto Field

Lomita Drive

Camino Alto

Vasco Drive

Azalea Drive

Birthedale Avenue

MILL VALLEY

Camino Alto

East Blithedale Avenue

Lomita Drive

101

Tiburon Boulevard

TIBURON

Sycamore Avenue

Harrison Skatepark

P

Mill Valley Community Center

Hauke Park

Hamilton Drive

Redwood Highway

Ricardo Road

Richardson Drive

Miller Avenue

P

Bayfront Park

Almonte Boulevard

Pickleweed Inlet

Bothin Marsh Preserve

STRAWBERRY POINT

101

Coyote Creek

Shoreline Highway   1

1

Richardson Bay

houseboat community

Donahue Street

Golden Gate National Recreation Area

MARIN CITY

101

MLK Park

Coloma Street

Harbor Drive

FINISH

Bridgeway

SAUSALITO

Spring Street

N

rails·to·trails
conservancy

0   0.25   0.5 mile

San Francisco

CALIFORNIA

Los Angeles

The Mill Valley/Sausalito Multiuse Pathway connects two culturally rich communities on the north side of the San Francisco Bay. In fact, it's the only way for folks on foot to get from one town to the other. It's also part of a developing 2,600-miles-plus Bay Area regional trail network being spearheaded by the Bay Area Trails Collaborative (**railsto trails.org/bay-area**) and Rails-to-Trails Conservancy as a TrailNation™ project to increase safe walking, biking, and trail access for millions of Bay Area residents.

The 3.7-mile trail is mostly paved, with a few wooden bridges over marshes and inlets, as well as a gravel shoulder used by equestrians. There are numerous connections to trailside parks and open spaces, such as Bayfront Park and the 112-acre Bothin Marsh Preserve. There aren't many trees along the trail, so be prepared to be out in the sun. Bike-commuter traffic can be heavy at times, and a segment passes alongside noisy US 101. The Sausalito waterfront and terminal for the Sausalito–San Francisco Ferry is less than a mile south of the southern end of the trail, making for a popular weekend excursion.

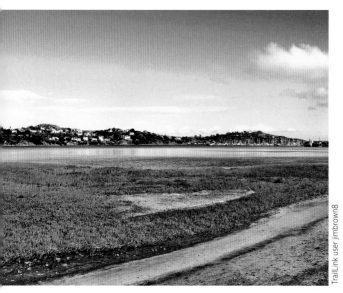
TrailLink user jimbrown8

The trail offers connections to parks and open spaces, such as the Bothin Marsh Preserve.

County
Marin

Endpoints
0.2 mile north of Vasco Ct. and Underhill Road (Mill Valley); Harbor Dr. and Bridgeway (Sausalito)

Mileage
3.7

Type
Rail-Trail

Roughness Rating
2

Surface
Asphalt

The trail follows the former route of the Mill Valley–Sausalito branch of the Northwestern Pacific Railroad, which ran more than 300 miles from San Rafael to the redwood forests of Humboldt County after its formation in the early 20th century. Passenger service was discontinued in 1940, and the pathway came into being in the 1970s. Long-range plans call for transforming the entire railroad corridor into the Great Redwoods Trail from San Rafael to Arcata.

Trail parking is located at Bayfront Park at the intersection with Sycamore Avenue, or you can find street parking. From the trail's north end in Mill Valley, you'll pass Alto Field and roll behind houses to a commercial area on East Blithedale Avenue. In 0.3 mile, you'll come to an unnamed trail intersection heading west to the town center or east to Hauke Park. Continuing south, you'll pass Harrison Skatepark and Bayfront Park on Pickleweed Inlet.

Crossing a bridge, the next 0.8 mile takes you through the Bothin Marsh Preserve, a destination for birders, as hundreds of bird species stop here during migratory seasons. Many ducks, gulls, and egrets make their year-round home in the tidal wetlands, as do marine mammals.

Immediately after crossing a bridge over Coyote Creek, you'll pass a trail heading west toward Sausalito. Heading southeast, you'll stay on the multiuse path, pass under US 101, and trace Richardson Bay and its houseboat community, made famous by those seeking an alternative lifestyle since the 1920s. The trail ends at Harbor Drive, although sidewalks run alongside Bridgeway for 1.6 miles to the Sausalito Ferry.

CONTACT rtc.li/marin-county-parks

PARKING

Parking areas are located within Mill Valley and are listed from north to south. *Indicates that at least one accessible parking space is available.*

MILL VALLEY COMMUNITY CENTER* 180 Camino Alto (37.8998, -122.5278).
BAYFRONT PARK* 499 Sycamore Ave. (37.8969, -122.5269).

The Mission Bay Bike Path forms an 11-mile, heart-shaped loop around San Diego's Mission Bay and the incredibly scenic 4,235-acre Mission Bay Park. The trail is part of the developing California Coastal Trail—a network of bicycling and hiking trails that, when complete, will stretch along the coastline for 1,230 miles from Oregon to the Mexican border.

Beginning from the bottom of the "heart," you'll find ample parking and restrooms at South Shores Park, just east of SeaWorld theme park. Heading east from the park, the paved pathway is a postcard-perfect snapshot of Southern California—broad, easy to navigate, and dotted with palm trees and wildflowers. Within a quick 0.1 mile, you'll hit your first bayside beach!

Continuing north, the designated path ends briefly at East Mission Bay Drive; turn left and follow the broad sidewalk past Fiesta Island Road, where the pathway begins

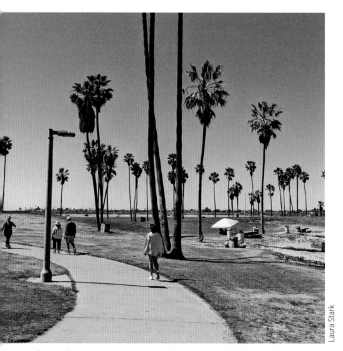

Laura Stark

Connecting numerous parks, the trail is dotted with playgrounds, picnic areas, and other amenities.

County
San Diego

Endpoint
South Shores Park at South Shores Pkwy., 0.2 mile west of Sea World Dr. (San Diego)

Mileage
11.4

Type
Greenway/Non-Rail-Trail

Roughness Rating
1

Surface
Asphalt, Concrete

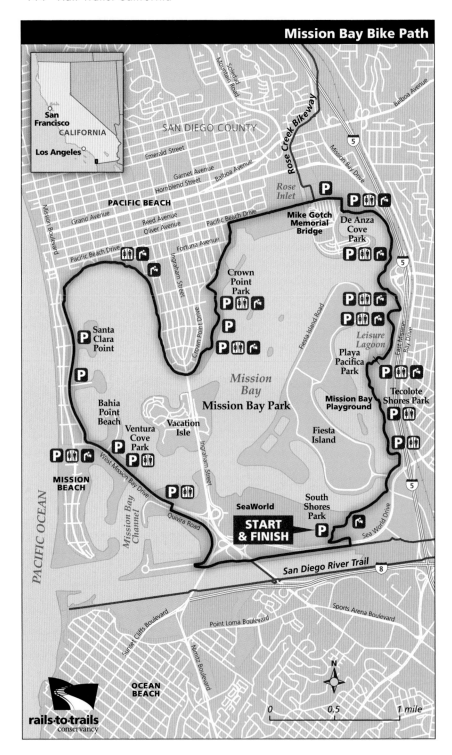

Mission Bay Bike Path

anew. You'll have the sparkling bay to your left and East Mission Bay Drive to your right. In 0.8 mile, you'll reach the sprawling Mission Bay Playground, its adjacent beach, and a broad grassy area perfect for picnics. The pleasant route then passes Tecolote Shores Park, Playa Pacifica Park, and the beaches along Leisure Lagoon in quick succession.

Rounding the eastern lobe of the "heart," you'll travel through De Anza Cove Park, which offers plentiful recreational amenities, including volleyball courts, covered picnic tables, and outdoor exercise equipment. The trail ends at this park's southwest corner, so you'll need to travel a short distance (0.3 mile) on-road: Turn right (north) onto De Anza Road, and then turn left (west) onto North Mission Bay Drive. The trail resumes its off-road nature at the Mike Gotch Memorial Bridge over the Rose Inlet; note that there is a slight incline as you approach the bridge.

After 0.4 mile, the trail empties out onto Pacific Beach Drive, a quiet residential road. Travel on-road 0.3 mile, then turn left (south) on Crown Point Drive through a neighborhood overlooking a coastal marsh; use caution, as there is no bike lane or bike route signage and only a narrow sidewalk. After 0.4 mile, you'll reach a fork in the road; veer left on Corona Oriente Road. In another 0.1 mile, you'll arrive at Crown Point Park and be reunited with the paved pathway.

The bike path loops around Mission Bay for just over 11 miles.   Laura Stark

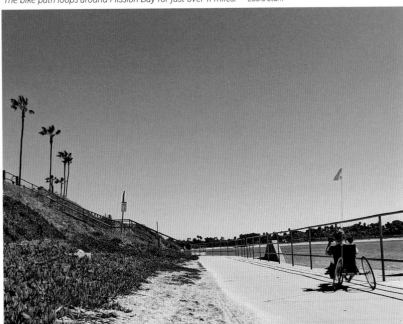

Following the Mission Bay shoreline, you'll have outstanding views and access to more beaches (so close that the trail becomes dusted with sand). Tracing the western lobe of the heart-shaped pathway, the route becomes increasingly crowded as you enter a lively destination area with numerous hotels and beautiful beachfront residences. When the path reaches West Mission Bay Drive, it's a good place to end your adventure, as the route becomes largely on-road from here, with limited trail signage.

If you wish to continue, follow the on-road bike lane southeast along West Mission Bay Drive. In 0.3 mile, you'll pass Ventura Cove Park and then cross the bridge over the Mission Bay Channel; be aware that the approach to the bridge involves a steep climb. At the end of the bridge, take a right to access Quivira Road at the first traffic light. Follow Quivira Road/Quivira Way southeast 0.7 mile until you see a paved path on your left marked with a small white BIKE PATH sign located opposite the parking lot for boat docks C–J. This trail entrance is easy to miss, so look for the large dirt parking lot adjacent to the trail.

The pathway will quickly head under a bridge (Sunset Cliffs Boulevard) and become on-road once more after passing under a second bridge (West Mission Bay Drive), but the road is a frontage road with very little traffic. Continue east 1.2 miles until you reach a traffic light for South Shores Parkway; turn left, crossing Sea World Drive, and follow the parkway back to your starting point at South Shores Park.

CONTACT rtc.li/mission-bay-bike-path

PARKING

Parking areas are located within San Diego and are listed counterclockwise, beginning at South Shores Park. Select parking areas for the trail are listed below. For a detailed list of parking areas and other waypoints, go to **TrailLink.com™**. *Indicates that at least one accessible parking space is available.*

SOUTH SHORES PARK* South Shores Pkwy., 0.2 mile west of Sea World Dr. (32.7629, -117.2181).

TECOLOTE SHORES PARK* 1740 E. Mission Bay Dr. (32.7756, -117.2099).

PLAYA PACIFICA PARK* 1093 E. Mission Bay Dr. (32.7810, -117.2110).

DE ANZA BOAT LAUNCH* 3500 Mission Bay Dr. (32.7930, -117.2087).

DE ANZA COVE* 3000 N. Mission Bay Dr. (32.7978, -117.2149).

CROWN POINT PARK* Corona Oriente Road and Moorland Dr. (32.7888, -117.2334).

SANTA CLARA RECREATION CENTER* 1008 Santa Clara Pl. (32.7829, -117.2505).

BONITA COVE* 1100 W. Mission Bay Dr. (32.7716, -117.2495).

VENTURA COVE PARK* 3209 Gleason Road (32.7698, -117.2440).

The Monterey Bay Coastal Recreation Trail offers breathtaking views of the Central Coast and an opportunity to explore Monterey and the nearby seaside towns of Pacific Grove, Seaside, Sand City, and Marina, as well as the farming community of Castroville.

Extending for 18 miles, the rail-trail provides many access points to the beach and is part of two developing coastal trail systems, the Monterey Bay Sanctuary Scenic Trail, which will trace the shoreline for some 50 miles to Wilder Ranch State Park north of Santa Cruz, and the California Coastal Trail, a network of bicycling and hiking trails that, when complete, will stretch along the coastline for 1,230 miles from Oregon to the Mexican border.

Much of the Monterey Bay Coastal Recreation Trail follows the corridor of the Southern Pacific Railroad's Monterey Branch. Launched in 1879, it served lumberyards in Pacific Grove, fish canneries and a swank hotel in Monterey, and productive vegetable farms in the Salinas Valley. Monterey County opened the trail in the mid-1980s.

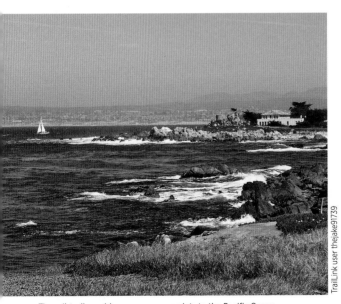

The rail-trail provides many access points to the Pacific Ocean.

TrailLink user thejake91739

County
Monterey

Endpoints
Jewell Ave. and Ocean View Blvd. (Pacific Grove); Haro St., 0.2 mile south of Merritt St./ CA 183 (Castroville)

Mileage
18

Type
Rail-Trail

Roughness Rating
1

Surface
Asphalt, Concrete

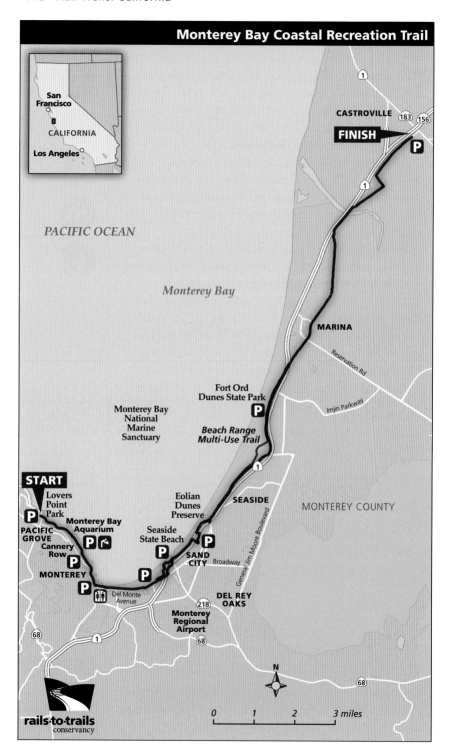

Monterey Bay Coastal Recreation Trail

The recreational trail extends along the edge of the Monterey Bay National Marine Sanctuary, which is home to such marine mammals as sea lions, dolphins, and whales, as well as hundreds of shorebird and fish species.

In the south, the trail starts at a rocky overlook at Pacific Grove's Lovers Point Park. The beach here draws sunbathers, as well as surfers, kayakers, and scuba divers. The south end of the trail can be congested at times, so watch for signage regarding lane usage and speed limits.

In a mile you'll come to Monterey's Cannery Row, a tourist destination that's nothing like the bars, marine labs, and fish canneries that inspired author John Steinbeck. Today, the waterfront street offers shopping, lodging, bike rentals, and entertainment for all ages. Steps from the trail, the local highlight is the Monterey Bay Aquarium, where local aquatic creatures, such as octopi, sea turtles, and sharks, swim in giant glass tanks.

Over the next 1.5 miles, you'll pass many businesses and three piers. The second one, Old Fishermen's Wharf, is the most touristy, while the others cater to the commercial and recreational fishing fleet docked nearby. The trail hugs the coast and climbs a dune (take the left fork 1.9 miles after the wharf) on the way into aptly named Sand City. The mountains of sand at Eolian Dunes Preserve occasionally drift onto the trail.

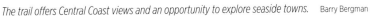

The trail offers Central Coast views and an opportunity to explore seaside towns. Barry Bergman

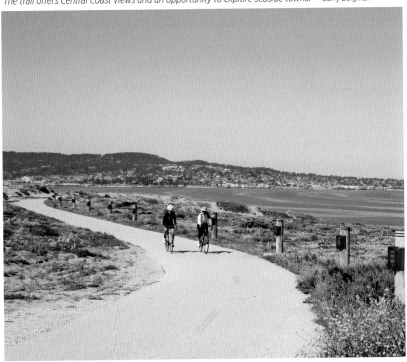

The trail runs alongside CA 1/Cabrillo Highway between the towns of Sand City and Marina. In Sand City, you'll take a 0.4-mile detour by turning right onto Tioga Avenue and then left onto Metz Road before turning left (at Playa Avenue) to return to the trail.

Proceeding north for 3 miles, you'll pass into Fort Ord Dunes State Park, once the site of an Army post. An alternative 4-mile route through the old base is the Beach Range Multi-Use Trail, reached at a trail junction 0.5 mile past the California Avenue intersection.

In Marina, the trail veers inland and runs alongside Del Monte Boulevard for 3.4 miles. It then veers right onto Monte Road and shares the roadway for 2 miles past Salinas Valley's vegetable farms. A left turn onto Nashua Road puts you back onto off-road trail for the remaining 1.7 miles to Castroville, known as the artichoke center of the world and celebrated in an annual June festival.

CONTACT rtc.li/city-of-monterey and rtc.li/city-of-pacific-grove

PARKING

Parking areas are listed from west to east. Select parking areas for the trail are listed below. For a detailed list of parking areas and other waypoints, go to **TrailLink.com™**. *Indicates that at least one accessible parking space is available.*

PACIFIC GROVE* Ocean View Blvd. and Jewell Ave. (36.6247, -121.9172).

MONTEREY* 501 Cannery Row (36.6143, -121.8991); paid parking.

MONTEREY* Fishermen's Wharf, 300 feet north of Del Monte Ave. (36.6012, -121.8902); paid parking.

MONTEREY* 588 Del Monte Blvd. (36.6001, -121.8875).

MONTEREY* 1949 Del Monte Ave. (36.6002, -121.8745).

SEASIDE* Seaside State Beach, Canyon Del Rey Blvd. and Sand Dunes Dr. (36.6114, -121.8576).

SAND CITY* Metz Road and Playa Ave. (36.6197, -121.8461).

SEASIDE* Fort Ord Dunes State Park, Eighth St. and Stilwell Hall (36.6605, -121.8211), about 0.4 mile west of First Ave.

CASTROVILLE Haro St., 0.2 mile south of Merritt St. (36.7594, -121.7547).

The path of an old tourist railway rolls through dizzying heights in the mountains near Pasadena in Southern California. Visitors are rewarded with inspiring views of rugged mountains, canyons, and the urban landscape below and can inspect ruins of mountaintop resorts and the remains of the railway.

Unlike the mostly smooth, straight routes followed by typical rail-trails, the Mt. Lowe Railway Trail clings to canyon sides as it meanders through the San Gabriel Mountains in the Angeles National Forest. Carry plenty of food and water, as neither is available on this trail.

Scientist and inventor Thaddeus S.C. Lowe created the railway as a tourist destination in the 1890s. It made a 2,200-foot ascent up Rubio Canyon from Altadena on a 62% grade achieved by using gears and counterbalanced passenger cars powered by electricity—the only such trolley in the country. Present-day visitors are spared

County
Los Angeles

Endpoints
Mt. Lowe Road Trailhead at Chaney Trl. and Brown Mountain Truck Trl. (Angeles National Forest); Mt. Lowe Trail Camp at Mt. Lowe Trail Road and Muir Peak Road (Angeles National Forest); White City resort ruins (Angeles National Forest)

Mileage
5.8

Type
Rail-Trail

Roughness Rating
2

Surface
Dirt, Gravel

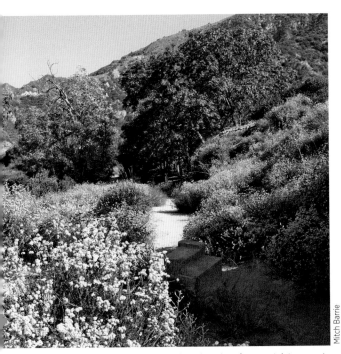

Mitch Barrie

Once a tourist railway, the route leads to the ruins of a mountaintop resort.

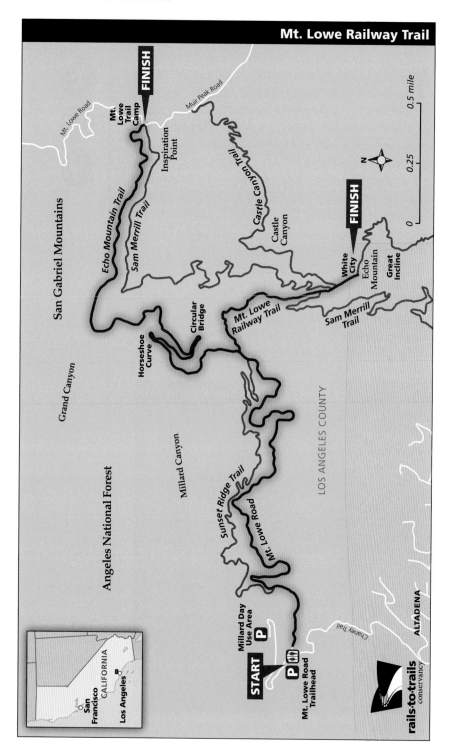

Mt. Lowe Railway Trail

FINISH

FINISH

San Gabriel Mountains

Angeles National Forest

Mt. Lowe Road

Muir Peak Road

Mt. Lowe Trail Camp

Inspiration Point

Echo Mountain Trail

Sam Merrill Trail

Castle Canyon Trail

Castle Canyon

White City

Echo Mountain

Great Incline

Mt. Lowe Railway Trail

Sam Merrill Trail

Circular Bridge

Horseshoe Curve

Grand Canyon

Millard Canyon

Sunset Ridge Trail

Mt. Lowe Road

LOS ANGELES COUNTY

Millard Day Use Area

START

Mt. Lowe Road Trailhead

Chaney Trail

ALTADENA

N

0   0.25   0.5 mile

CALIFORNIA

San Francisco

Los Angeles

rails-to-trails
conservancy

that climb up the Great Incline (which was demolished after the railway ceased operating in 1938) by starting their explorations from a trailhead on a roadway named Chaney Trail about a mile north of Altadena. Still, the route climbs about 1,400 feet to the ruins on Echo Mountain and 2,400 feet to Mt. Lowe Trail Camp.

Passing through the gate, you'll take Mt. Lowe Road, a fire road, 2.4 miles to reach the junction with the Mt. Lowe Railway Trail. Take the right fork onto the dirt trail, which leads to the ruins of the White City resort in 0.8 mile.

The resort included a 70-room, Victorian-style hotel, as well as an observatory, a casino, a dance hall, a zoo, and more. After Lowe went bankrupt, the Pacific Electric Railway acquired the operation. Along with a historical marker and artifacts from the railway, such as cars, wheels, and giant gears, you'll find foundations remaining for many buildings that were claimed by fire, landslides, and neglect over the years. Facing south, you'll have views of the Los Angeles Basin. (From here, the Sam Merrill Trail heads downhill to the Cobb Estate trailhead in Altadena and serves as an alternative way to reach the White City ruins.)

Returning to the trail junction, head right (north) onto Mount Lowe Road, which overlaps the Mt. Lowe Railway Trail and Echo Mountain Trail routes, to follow the old railway corridor's Alpine Division, which ran between White City and a tavern near Mount Lowe. Soon you'll negotiate the longest straight section of the railway route, spanning just 225 feet. This leads to two tight switchbacks, the first called Horseshoe Curve and the second, Circular Bridge, the site of a wooden trestle suspended over the canyon below.

The trail continues along a mountainside overlooking Millard and Grand Canyons for nearly 3 miles to Mt. Lowe Trail Camp, the former site of Ye Alpine Tavern, a Swiss chalet–style hotel that served guests from 1895 to 1936. Guests could walk 0.4 mile south to Inspiration Point, which still exists, for views of the Catalina Islands. At 4,400 feet elevation, the tavern marked the terminus of the railway's Alpine Division.

CONTACT fs.usda.gov/recmain/angeles/recreation

PARKING

Parking areas are located within Angeles National Forest on the west end of the trail; no parking lots are available on the trail's east end. *Indicates that at least one accessible parking space is available.*

MT. LOWE ROAD TRAILHEAD Chaney Trl. and Brown Mountain Truck Trl., 1.2 mile north of W. Loma Vista Dr. (34.2148, -118.1478).

MILLARD DAY USE AREA* Chaney Trl. and Brown Mountain Truck Trl., 1.7 mile north of W. Loma Vista Dr. (34.2163, -118.1465).

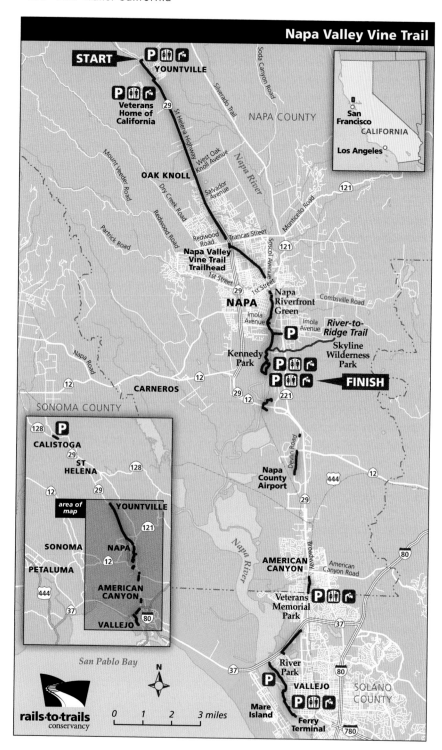

Napa Valley Vine Trail

START
YOUNTVILLE

Veterans
Home of
California

Soda Canyon Road

Silverado Trail

NAPA COUNTY

San
Francisco

CALIFORNIA

Los Angeles

29

Napa River

121

OAK KNOLL

West Oak
Knoll Avenue

Mount Veeder Road

Dry Creek Road

Redwood Road

St Helena Highway

Salvador
Avenue

Monticello Road

Partrick Road

Redwood
Road

Trancas Street

Napa Valley
Vine Trail
Trailhead

Soscol Avenue

121

1st Street

29   1st Street

NAPA

Napa
Riverfront
Green

Combsville Road

Imola
Avenue

Imola
Avenue

River-to-
Ridge Trail

Napa Road

Kennedy
Park

Skyline
Wilderness
Park

12

12

CARNEROS

SONOMA COUNTY

29

12

221

FINISH

128

P

CALISTOGA

29

ST
HELENA

128

12

29

area of
map

YOUNTVILLE

121

SONOMA

NAPA

12

PETALUMA

444

AMERICAN
CANYON

37

VALLEJO

80

Devlin Road

Napa
County
Airport

444

12

29

Napa River

AMERICAN
CANYON

Broadway

American
Canyon Road

80

Veterans
Memorial
Park

P

37

San Pablo Bay

N

River
Park

P

VALLEJO

37

P

SOLANO
COUNTY

80

Mare
Island

Ferry
Terminal

780

rails·to·trails
conservancy

0   1   2   3 miles

The Napa Valley Vine Trail is a wine lover's dream, as it will eventually roll down the center of California's trendy North Coast winery region for 47 miles. It will pass wide swaths of vineyards and dozens of wineries from its northern end at the mud baths in Calistoga to the ferry terminal just off San Pablo Bay in Vallejo. As of 2023, there are about 18.5 miles of paved trail segments in Calistoga, Napa, American Canyon, and Vallejo, and completion is slated for the middle of the decade.

As of spring 2023, the endpoints for completed sections are as follows:

➤ Washington St. at Tedeschi Field, 0.1 mile east of Camp Dr. (Calistoga); Dunaweal Lane, 1 mile north of CA 29/St. Helena Hwy. (Calistoga)

➤ Madison St. and Washington St. (Yountville); Vallejo St. and Soscol Ave. (Napa)

➤ Third St. and Soscol Ave. (Napa); John F. Kennedy Memorial Park at Streblow Dr. (Napa)

➤ Anselmo Ct., 0.2 mile west of Napa Valley Corporate Dr. (Napa); Soscol Ferry Road, 0.3 mile west of Napa Valley Corporate Dr.

Counties
Napa, Solano

Endpoints
Northernmost: Washington St. at Tedeschi Field, 0.1 mile east of Camp Dr. (Calistoga) *Southernmost:* Vallejo Launch Ramp at Curtola Pkwy., 0.1 mile south of Maine St. (Vallejo). *Full list of endpoints in text.*

Mileage
18.5

Type
Rail-Trail/Rail-with-Trail

Roughness Rating
1

Surface
Asphalt, Concrete, Crushed Stone

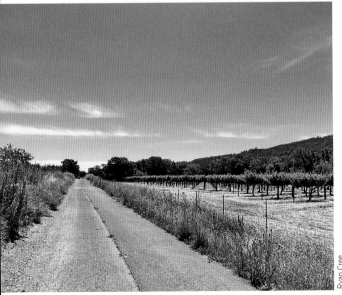

Ryan Cree

Napa Valley vineyards and wineries are frequent sights along the trail.

➤ Airport Blvd. and Devlin Road (Napa); Tower Road and Devlin Road (American Canyon)

➤ Veterans Memorial Park at Broadway/Lincoln Hwy., 0.2 mile south of W. American Canyon Road (American Canyon); Broadway/Lincoln Hwy. and Vine Terrace Way (American Canyon)

➤ Sonoma Blvd. and Lewis Brown Dr. (Vallejo); Sacramento St., 0.1 mile east of CA 37 (Vallejo)

➤ Wilson Ave. and CA 37/Sears Point Road (Vallejo); Vallejo Launch Ramp at Curtola Pkwy., 0.1 mile south of Maine St. (Vallejo)

The trail follows the route of the old Napa Valley Railroad, which was completed in the 1860s to take tourists from the docks in Vallejo to the resort in Calistoga. Later sold, the rail corridor closed in the 1980s, but the section between Napa and Calistoga was revived by the new Napa Valley Railroad, which offers multiple dinner-train excursions daily.

The trail south of Napa is part of the 500-mile San Francisco Bay Trail network, while a short segment in the north is part of the 550-mile Bay Area Ridge Trail network. All are part of a developing 2,600-miles-plus Bay Area regional trail network being spearheaded by the Bay Area Trails Collaborative (**railsto trails.org/bay-area**) and Rails-to-Trails Conservancy as a TrailNation™ project to increase safe walking, biking, and trail access for millions of Bay Area residents.

The longest stretch of the Napa Valley Vine Trail—12 miles—runs from Yountville to John F. Kennedy Park in Napa. Heading south from Madison Street in Yountville, a town known for its delicious dining and sparkling wines,

Between Napa and Calistoga, you'll share the corridor with the Napa Valley Railroad.   Joe LaCroix

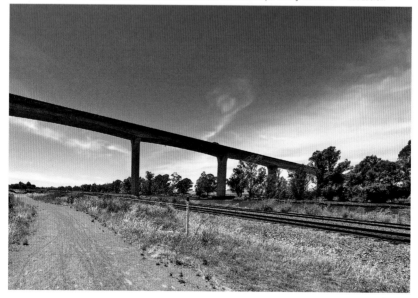

you'll cross to the west side of CA 29/St. Helena Highway in 0.8 mile at the historic Veterans Home of California. You're soon immersed in the Napa Valley viticulture as you frequently pass vineyards and wineries on a corridor shared with the highway and the excursion train.

The vineyards end in 3.8 miles as you enter Napa, which features more dining, parks, and wine tasting rooms. The path is interrupted in 2.2 miles at the Napa Valley Vine Trail Trailhead at Redwood Road and Solano Avenue. Cross Redwood Road and head east for a half block to resume the trail, which crosses CA 29 on an overpass.

After traveling through residential and light industrial areas for 1.7 miles, the trail breaks again at Vallejo Street. To reach the end of the trail in Kennedy Park, head east for a half block on Vallejo Street and follow the sidewalk south on Soscol Avenue 0.8 mile, passing the excursion train station along the way. Cross the Napa River, or head west on First Avenue for a side trip into Napa's dining and boutique district. One block past the river, pick up the trail heading south at the Napa Riverfront Green. The trail flows along the river for 2.5 miles to the 350-acre Kennedy Park, where it meets the River-to-Ridge Trail. The segment ends just past the skate park and baseball fields.

New sections of trail are rolling out regularly, with a segment linking Calistoga with St. Helena slated to open in 2023.

CONTACT vinetrail.org

PARKING

Parking areas are listed from north to south. Select parking areas for the trail are listed below. For a detailed list of parking areas and other waypoints, go to **TrailLink.com™**. *Indicates that at least one accessible parking space is available.*

CALISTOGA Little League–Tedeschi Field, 304 Washington St. (38.5765, -122.5711).

YOUNTVILLE* Veterans Home Trailhead, California Dr. and Solano Ave. (38.3971, -122.3596).

NAPA* Kennedy Park, 2295 Streblow Dr. (38.2687, -122.2827).

AMERICAN CANYON* Veterans Memorial Park, 2800 Lincoln Hwy./Broadway (38.1628, -122.2520).

VALLEJO* River Park, Wilson Ave./Mare Island Way and Hichborn St. (38.1129, -122.2672).

VALLEJO* Ferry Terminal Parking (fees charged), Mare Island Way and Georgia St. (38.1009, -122.2632).

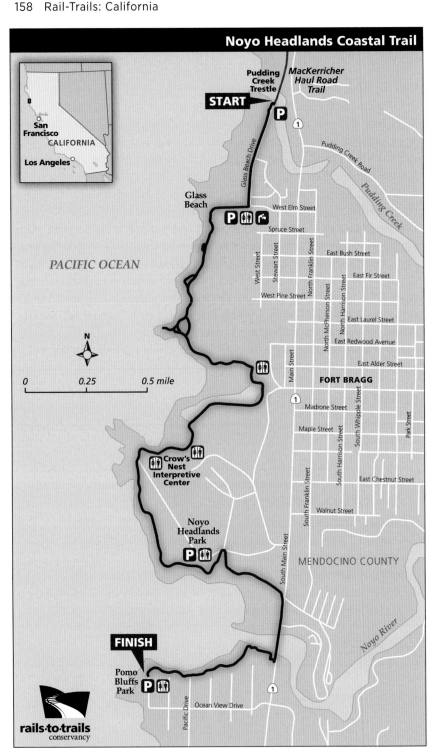

Noyo Headlands Coastal Trail

Pudding Creek Trestle

MacKerricher Haul Road Trail

START

P

1

Glass Beach Drive

Pudding Creek Road

Pudding Creek

San Francisco

CALIFORNIA

Los Angeles

Glass Beach

P

West Elm Street

Spruce Street

West Street

Stewart Street

North Franklin Street

East Bush Street

East Fir Street

PACIFIC OCEAN

West Pine Street

North McPherson Street

North Harrison Street

East Laurel Street

East Redwood Avenue

N

East Alder Street

Main Street

FORT BRAGG

1

Madrone Street

South Whipple Street

Park Street

0   0.25   0.5 mile

Maple Street

South Harrison Street

East Chestnut Street

Crow's Nest Interpretive Center

South Franklin Street

Walnut Street

Noyo Headlands Park

P

MENDOCINO COUNTY

South Main Street

Noyo River

FINISH

Pomo Bluffs Park

P

1

Pacific Drive

Ocean View Drive

rails·to·trails
conservancy

ocated west of downtown Fort Bragg, the Noyo Headlands Coastal Trail transformed this former Georgia Pacific Railway mill site into a place for enjoying expansive views of the Pacific Ocean. The paved 4.5-mile pathway provides dawn-to-dusk access to the area's rugged clifftops and beaches. If you time it right, you might even see whales migrating during your excursion. It's also one of the newest segments of the California Coastal Trail, a network of bicycling and hiking trails that, when complete, will stretch along the coastline for 1,230 miles from Oregon to the Mexican border.

Begin on the trail's north end and visit the historical Pudding Creek Trestle spanning just over 500 feet across a beach. For more than a century, Fort Bragg was known for its sawmills until the last of them closed in 2002. Railroads were used to speed up the logging process, and the

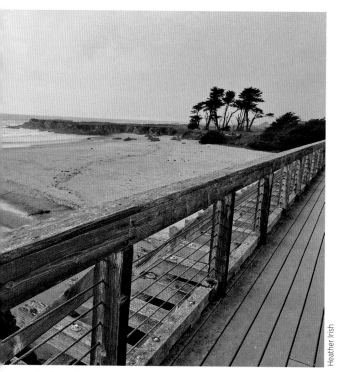

On the trail's north end, visit the historical Pudding Creek Trestle.

Heather Irish

County
Mendocino

Endpoints
Dead end of Glass Beach Dr., 0.4 mile north of W. Elm St. (Fort Bragg); Pomo Bluffs Park at the dead end of Cliff Way, 0.1 mile north of Ocean View Dr. (Fort Bragg)

Mileage
4.5

Type
Greenway/Non-Rail-Trail

Roughness Rating
1

Surface
Asphalt

route of the Ten Mile Railroad, completed in 1916, included the Pudding Creek Trestle. At the bridge, the trail connects to the MacKerricher Haul Road Trail (see page 127), which follows the former timber-hauling rail line north along the coastline and reaches MacKerricher State Park.

Head south from the bridge to experience the Noyo Headlands Coastal Trail. In 0.5 mile, you'll reach the parking lot for Glass Beach, named for the small pieces of smoothed glass that cover the sand. Continuing your journey along the coast, you'll find a scenic overlook in 0.7 mile with a compass rose artwork set into the ground. Another 1.1 miles will bring you to the Crow's Nest Interpretive Center, which offers a tidepool aquarium and marine mammal exhibits. After 2.2 miles, you'll arrive at the 25-acre Pomo Bluffs Park and the end of the trail.

There are several restrooms along the path, including an artistically tiled facility that includes a bike repair station, located near the trail's midpoint. Local artisans have also created a variety of unique benches.

Interpretative panels along the path educate visitors on environmental and historical topics. The many footpaths to the bluffs allow for close-up encounters with wildflowers and the captivating terrain. Along this route, keep an eye out for endangered flowers that inhabit the area: the bright-yellow Point Reyes blennosperma, the fiery-red Mendocino Coast paintbrush, and the white-blossomed Howell's spineflower.

CONTACT rtc.li/city-fort-bragg

PARKING

Parking areas listed are located within Fort Bragg and are listed from north to south. *Indicates that at least one accessible parking space is available.*

PUDDING CREEK TRESTLE* Dead end of Glass Beach Dr., 0.4 mile north of W. Elm St. (39.4577, -123.8080).

GLASS BEACH* Glass Beach Dr. and Noyo Point Road (39.4519, -123.8104).

NOYO HEADLANDS PARK* Noyo Point Road and W. Cypress St. (39.4316, -123.8127).

POMO BLUFFS PARK* 19301 Cliff Way (39.4254, -123.8163).

The Ohlone Greenway waltzes through the Bay Area cities of Berkeley, Albany, and El Cerrito for 5.3 miles with its partner, Bay Area Rapid Transit (BART). Doubling as a commuter and recreation route through the urban setting, the trail is named for the Indigenous people who once lived throughout Central California's coastal areas. It's also part of a developing 2,600-miles-plus Bay Area regional trail network being spearheaded by the Bay Area Trails Collaborative (**railstotrails.org/bay-area**) and Rails-to-Trails Conservancy as a TrailNation™ project to increase safe walking, biking, and trail access for millions of Bay Area residents.

The paved trail links several parks and community gardens, as well as business districts with opportunities for refreshments. The ever-present elevated BART tracks lead to three stations, where bicyclists and walkers can board trains to destinations anywhere on the 130-mile system (see **bart.gov/guide/bikes**).

The greenway right-of-way dates back to the 1880s, when it was a transportation corridor for several railroads.

Counties
Alameda, Contra Costa

Endpoints
Martin Luther King Jr. Way and Hearst Ave. (Berkeley); Richmond Greenway and San Pablo Ave., 190 feet north of Ohio St. (El Cerrito)

Mileage
5.3

Type
Rail-with-Trail

Roughness Rating
1

Surface
Asphalt

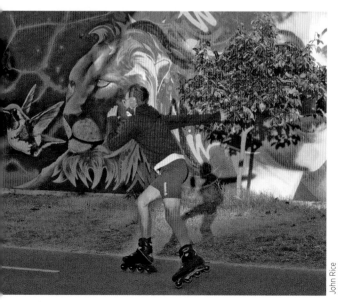

Serving as a linear park, the trail hosts public art, a community garden, and other attractions.

John Rice

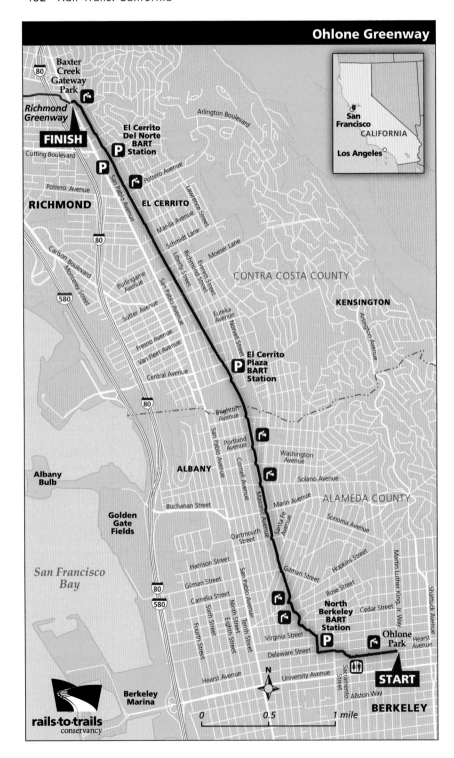

Ohlone Greenway

Baxter Creek Gateway Park

Richmond Greenway

FINISH

Cutting Boulevard

RICHMOND

Potrero Avenue

El Cerrito Del Norte BART Station

Potrero Avenue

EL CERRITO

Arlington Boulevard

Lawrence Street

Manila Avenue

Schmidt Lane

Liberty Street

Richmond Street

Everett Street

Moeser Lane

CONTRA COSTA COUNTY

KENSINGTON

Arlington Avenue

San Pablo Avenue

Burlingame Avenue

Sutter Avenue

Fresno Avenue

Van Fleet Avenue

Central Avenue

Eureka Avenue

Norvell Street

El Cerrito Plaza BART Station

Brighton Avenue

Portland Avenue

San Pablo Avenue

Cornell Avenue

Washington Avenue

Solano Avenue

ALBANY

Buchanan Street

Marin Avenue

Santa Fe Avenue

Masonic Avenue

ALAMEDA COUNTY

Sonoma Avenue

Albany Bulb

Golden Gate Fields

Dartmouth Street

Harrison Street

Gilman Street

Camelia Street

Sixth Street

Ninth Street

Eighth Street

Tenth Street

San Pablo Avenue

Gilman Street

Hopkins Street

Rose Street

Cedar Street

Martin Luther King, Jr. Way

Shattuck Avenue

San Francisco Bay

Fourth Street

Virginia Street

North Berkeley BART Station

Delaware Street

Hearst Avenue

Ohlone Park

Hearst Avenue

Sacramento Street

START

University Avenue

Allston Way

Berkeley Marina

BERKELEY

rails·to·trails conservancy

0   0.5   1 mile

N

San Francisco
CALIFORNIA
Los Angeles

One of these, the Key System, rolled through Berkeley to the San Francisco Bay ferry crossing in Emeryville. Separately, the California & Mt. Diablo Railroad ran through the corridor on narrow-gauge tracks laid in the 1880s. Eventually, the Atchison, Topeka and Santa Fe Railway (often referred to as Santa Fe) gained control in 1903 and widened the tracks to handle commonly sized freight cars running between Richmond and Oakland. Santa Fe stopped using the tracks in the late 1970s.

The trail starts in the south at linear Ohlone Park, which is situated along four blocks of Hearst Avenue, in one of Berkeley's oldest neighborhoods, within a half mile of the University of California, Berkeley's campus. Initially slated for apartments in the incendiary late 1960s, the space was turned over to the city after activists planted sod and trees and set up camp in protest. You'll find an off-leash dog park (one of the nation's first), exercise equipment, a playground, and a community garden here.

The North Berkeley BART station complex interrupts the greenway after a half mile at Sacramento Street. To reach the off-road trail again, take Delaware Street one block west, turn north on Acton Street, go one block, and return to the trail at the northwest corner of Virginia and Acton Streets. (Separated bike lanes to connect the trail segments are scheduled to be installed through the BART complex by mid-2023.)

The greenway continues through neighborhoods and commercial areas in a northwesterly direction. Unlike the BART tracks passing overhead, the greenway is impeded by stops at frequent major street crossings. You'll find eateries and shopping at the Solano Avenue intersection in Albany, about 1.3 miles north of Berkeley.

After passing through Albany, the greenway arrives at the El Cerrito Plaza BART station in about a mile. It's another 2 miles through commercial and residential areas to the El Cerrito Del Norte BART station. The Ohlone Greenway ends in a half mile at Baxter Creek Gateway Park, where it seamlessly joins the 3-mile Richmond Greenway (see page 179).

CONTACT rtc.li/ohlone-greenway

continued on next page

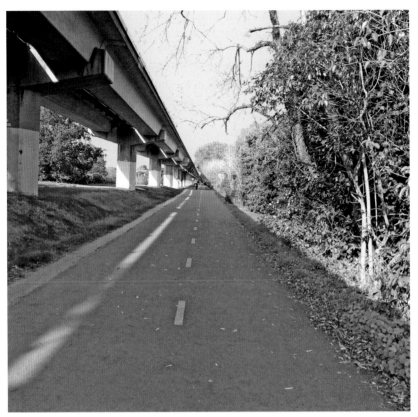

The Ohlone Greenway runs parallel to elevated BART tracks from Berkeley to El Cerrito.   Yoshi Oribe

PARKING

Parking areas are listed from south to north. *Indicates that at least one accessible parking space is available.*

BERKELEY* North Berkeley BART station, Delaware St. and Sacramento St. (37.8732, -122.2833); fee charged Monday–Friday, 4 a.m.–3 p.m.

EL CERRITO* El Cerrito Plaza BART station, Central Ave. and Liberty St. (37.9028, -122.2999); fee charged Monday–Friday, 4 a.m.–3 p.m.

EL CERRITO* El Cerrito Del Norte BART station, 6465 Hill St. (37.9247, -122.3174); fee charged Monday–Friday, 4 a.m.–3 p.m.

EL CERRITO* El Cerrito Del Norte BART station, Cutting Ave. and Key Blvd. (37.9259, -122.3163); fee charged Monday–Friday, 4 a.m.–3 p.m.

Street parking is available in Berkeley/Albany on Masonic Ave., between Santa Fe Ave. (37.883769, -122.2913) and Brighton Ave. (37.897603, -122.2958).

The Southern California town of Ojai (pronounced OH-hi) is known as a destination for wellness tourism, so it's fitting that those visiting via the Ojai Valley Trail are already practicing a healthy lifestyle. The 9.3-mile rail-trail climbs a river valley into the Topatopa Mountains from the outskirts of the seaside town of Ventura. It gains about 500 feet as it enters the Los Padres National Forest from the trailhead in Foster Park, where the Ventura River Trail (see page 239) heads downhill to the coast.

Two paths comprise the Ojai Valley Trail—one paved, one wood chips. They are separated by a fence to give horse riders a lane to themselves. The trail generally follows CA 33, the main route into Ojai, which is known as a haven for artists, musicians, and outdoors enthusiasts. The Chumash people were the first residents of the town, whose current name is derived from their word for moon: 'awha'y.

The trail follows the route of the former Ventura and Ojai Valley Railroad, which was launched in 1899. It soon became a branch of the Southern Pacific Railroad, which rolled through Ventura. Heavy rains in the winter of 1969 washed out the railbed north of Foster Park; trains never returned, and the trail opened in 1989.

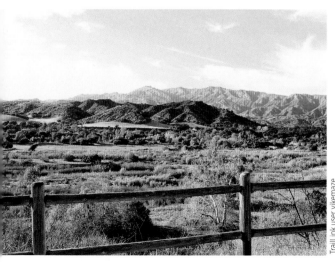

The scenic Ojai Valley Trail includes views of Los Padres National Forest and the Topatopa Mountains.

TrailLink user vikemaze

County
Ventura

Endpoints
Ventura River Trail at Casitas Vista Road, 0.1 mile west of N. Ventura Ave. (Foster Park); Bryant St., 0.1 mile south of Bryant Pl. (Ojai)

Mileage
9.3

Type
Rail-Trail

Roughness Rating
1

Surface
Asphalt, Wood Chips

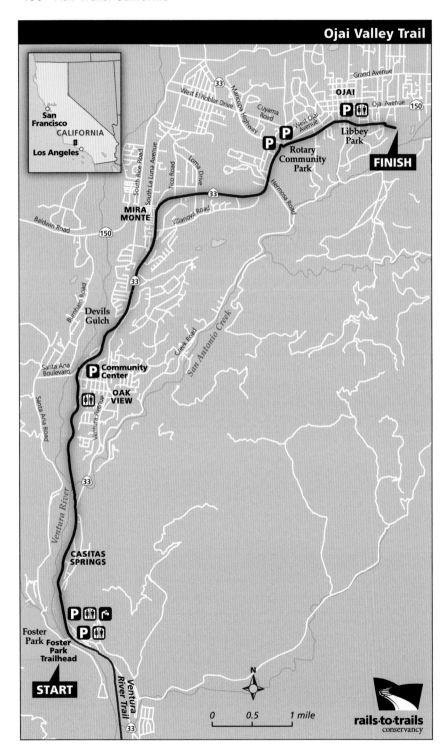

Ojai Valley Trail

The Foster Park trailhead has parking (for a nominal fee), restrooms, and a campground. It's located in a wooded valley alongside the Ventura River, where the Ojai Valley Trail and Ventura River Trail meet. The trail is mostly shady as you head north by CA 33 and pass through several communities.

The first of these is Casitas Springs (country musician Johnny Cash lived nearby for a time), which you'll pass in a mile. A bridge spanning San Antonio Creek a half mile north replaced a low-water creek crossing that occasionally got trail users wet. The trail veers west away from CA 33 for the next 3 miles as you pass the western side of Oak View, the largest community between Ventura and Ojai.

After a short excursion through Devils Gulch, known locally for its hiking trails, you'll find yourself back alongside CA 33 as you enter the community of Mira Monte. One mile past the busy CA 150/Baldwin Road intersection, you'll arrive in the town of Ojai. Crossing CA 33, you'll pass a sweeping golf course, spa, and resort complex on your right, and then in 0.3 mile, you'll pass the rear entrance (on your left) to Topa Mountain Winery, one of about half a dozen wineries or tasting rooms in the city.

In another 0.6 mile, you reach promised shade in Libbey Park, which offers parking, restrooms, a playground, and the Libbey Bowl amphitheater, site of early June's Ojai Music Festival. An easy path leads through the park to downtown Ojai, where you can explore many locally owned shops—chain stores are prohibited by law—in a setting reminiscent of a whitewashed hacienda. The trail ends a half mile past the park.

Closure Notice: Due to the 2022–2023 storms, a section of the Ojai Valley Trail is closed in Oak View between the San Antonio Creek Bridge and Prospect Street. Repairs are underway by the Ojai Valley Sanitation District; visit their website for details: **rtc.li/ovsd.**

CONTACT rtc.li/ojai-valley-trail

PARKING

Parking areas are listed from south to north. *Indicates that at least one accessible parking space is available.*

VENTURA* Foster Park, Ventura River Area entrance, 0.4 mile north of Casitas Vista Road (34.3568, -119.3097).

OAK VIEW* Community Center, 18 Valley Road (34.4020, -119.3036).

OJAI* N. Carillo Road and Maricopa Hwy. (34.4416, -119.2621); 2-hour parking, 9 a.m.–6 p.m.

OJAI* Rotary Community Park, 1199 W. Ojai Ave./CA 150 (34.4416, -119.2597).

OJAI* Libbey Park, 521 S. Montgomery St. (34.4448, -119.2439).

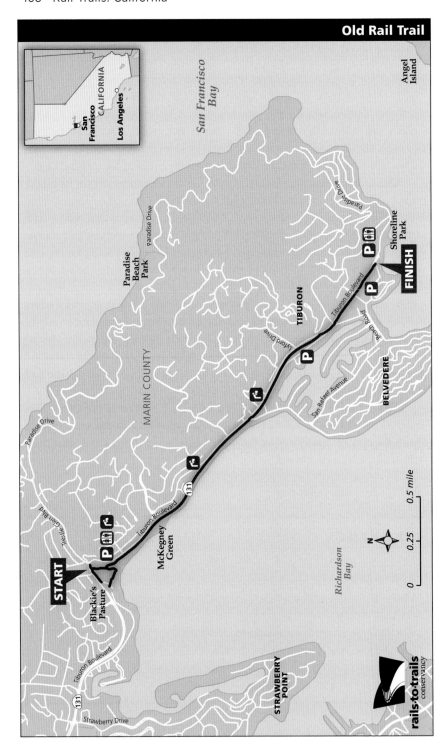

Old Rail Trail

If you're looking for a gentle rail-trail in Marin County that offers stunning views of both San Francisco Bay and Mount Tamalpais, the Old Rail Trail is for you. Also known as the Tiburon Historical Trail, Tiburon Bike Path, and Tiburon Linear Park, the trail begins at Blackie's Pasture, a scenic landing named after a celebrated, sway-backed, retired cavalry horse that once roamed here.

Heading south from Blackie's Pasture, you'll soon pass the coastal mudflats of Richardson Bay, a transition zone between land and sea that hosts a wide variety of plants and wildlife. A bird's (and birder's) paradise, the bay hosts more than 1 million migratory birds every year, along with a diverse mix of year-round avian residents, including great blue herons, snowy egrets, and red-tailed hawks. Breathtaking views of the bay start here and stay with you for the remainder of the trail.

The family-friendly rail-trail passes a number of playgrounds, small parks, and playing fields and is a great

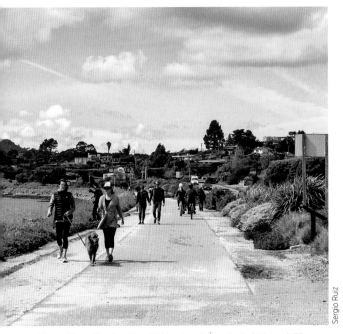

Sergio Ruiz

The trail hugs the shoreline of Richardson Bay as it winds through Tiburon.

County
Marin

Endpoints
Blackie's Pasture, just south of Tiburon Blvd. (Tiburon); Angel Island–Tiburon Ferry terminal on Main St. (Tiburon)

Mileage
2.6

Type
Rail-Trail

Roughness Rating
1

Surface
Asphalt

destination for a picnic or afternoon outing. It's also popular with cyclists and joggers, and with a paved section and wide dirt shoulder, there's ample room for both. The trail is relatively flat for most of its distance, with one gradual grade change early on near McKegney Green (about 0.5 mile from the northern endpoint), where the paved path connects to an upper path. That said, the trail is very easy to use for all ages and ability levels.

The trail runs along the coast through the town of Tiburon and into the city of Belvedere. Now among the most exclusive communities in the San Francisco Bay Area, both had humble beginnings. In the early 1900s, Tiburon was a blue-collar railroad town, with cargo trains running daily. One of the railroad's most famous "deliveries" was Al Capone, who was carried by train to nearby Alcatraz Island in 1934. Belvedere, meanwhile, once hosted an ever-pungent factory of the McCollam Fishing and Trading Company (now known as the Union Fish Company).

At about mile 2, the path becomes an on-street bike lane along Tiburon Boulevard/CA 131. Continue into downtown Tiburon and the trail's end at the ferry terminal by Shoreline Park. Here you'll find more great views of the bay, a host of restaurants and shops, a railroad and ferry depot museum, and the perfect spot to watch the sun set. The terminal is also a great launching point for more adventures: you can take a ferry to nearby Angel Island or San Francisco or continue along the Paradise Loop, a popular on-street route for cyclists.

The Old Rail Trail is a component of the San Francisco Bay Trail, an effort to create a 500-mile multiuse trail encircling the bay. The San Francisco Bay Trail, in turn, is part of a developing 2,600-miles-plus Bay Area regional trail network being spearheaded by the Bay Area Trails Collaborative (**railstotrails.org/bay -area**) and Rails-to-Trails Conservancy as a TrailNation™ project to increase safe walking, biking, and, trail access for millions of Bay Area residents.

CONTACT townoftiburon.org/201/public-works

PARKING

Parking areas are located within Tiburon and are listed from north to south. *Indicates that at least one accessible parking space is available.*

BLACKIE'S PASTURE* Blackie's Pasture, just south of Tiburon Blvd. (37.8962, -122.4904).

PUBLIC PARKING LOT* Tiburon Blvd., just south of Lyford Dr. (37.8797, -122.4644).

ANGEL ISLAND–TIBURON FERRY, MAIN STREET LOT* Main St., 0.1 mile west of Tiburon Blvd. (37.8734, -122.4572); for information on parking fees, visit **angelislandferry.com/parking-information.**

ANGEL ISLAND–TIBURON FERRY, POINT TIBURON LOT* Tiburon Blvd., east of the traffic circle (37.8743, -122.4546); cash-only lot. For information on parking fees, visit **angelislandferry.com/parking-information.**

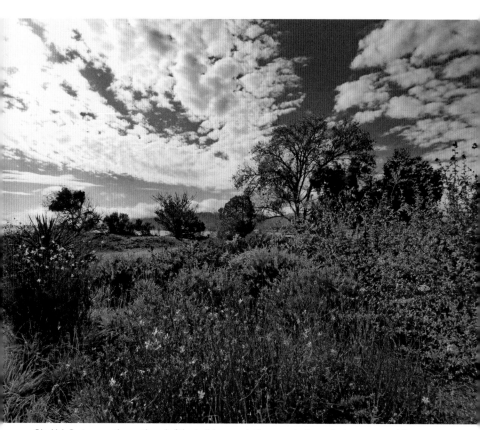

Blackie's Pasture, on the north end of the trail, is named after a cavalry horse that once roamed there.
Ginny Winblad

Old Railroad Grade

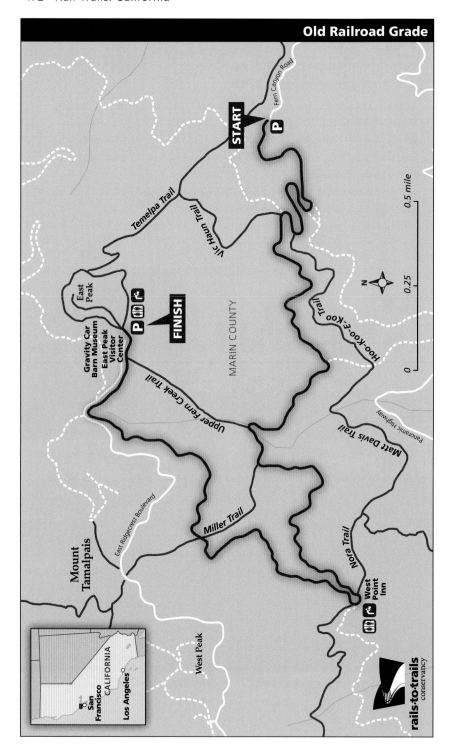

The view of the San Francisco Bay region from atop the East Peak of Mount Tamalpais is spectacular. Getting there on the 4.4-mile Old Railroad Grade can be just as impressive. The trail follows the route carved by the Mount Tamalpais and Muir Woods Railway, which opened in 1896 and soon became known as the Crookedest Railroad in the World. The railroad negotiated 281 curves and 22 trestles on its climb from the old depot that still stands in the heart of Mill Valley. Today, visitors start their ascent to the 2,571-foot summit from the end of Fern Valley Road and gain 1,309 feet of elevation from the trailhead. The packed-dirt route carries hikers, horseback riders, and mountain bikers (wide tires are recommended for the rough surface) to the top.

Railroad crews built the Mount Tamalpais Scenic Railroad in six months in 1896, and steam locomotives began regular runs carrying passengers up the mountain.

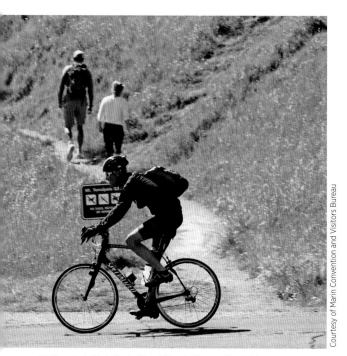

Mt. Tamalpais State Park offers hiking trails as well as biking opportunities on fire roads.

Courtesy of Marin Convention and Visitors Bureau

County
Marin

Endpoints
Fern Canyon Road,
0.6 mile west of Summit
Ave.; Mt. Tamalpais
State Park Visitor Center
(Mill Valley)

Mileage
4.4

Type
Rail-Trail

Roughness Rating
2

Surface
Dirt

Six years later, "Muir Woods" was added to the tourist railroad's name, as passengers could choose to make a return trip through the old-growth grove of coastal redwoods via so-called gravity cars, small four-wheel carts that whisked passengers downhill at 10–12 miles per hour. A devastating wildland fire that swept over Mount Tam spelled the end of the railroad in 1929; by then motorists had been driving to the summit via Ridgecrest Boulevard for four years. Today, a replica of a gravity car is housed in the Gravity Car Barn Museum at the summit.

Visitors can start at the roadside parking spots at the end of Fern Canyon Road. Take the right fork and pass through the gate across the trail, which also serves as a fire road into property controlled by the Marin Municipal Water District (the summit and adjacent land are part of Mt. Tamalpais State Park). You'll pass junctions with several hiking trails along the way; bicycles are only allowed on fire roads.

On the way to the East Peak, you will trek through areas of grassland and brushy chaparral, as well as stands of Douglas-fir and redwood. Hawks and turkey vultures are often seen soaring over the open spaces, while coyotes, bobcats, and raccoons prowl near the trail.

In 0.4 mile, you'll begin following the "double bow knot," where the railroad builders zigzagged four times to gain elevation up the mountainside. At 2.7 miles from the trail entrance, you'll come to West Point Inn, a lodge with dramatic views that dates to 1904 as a railway stop. It still hosts guests, who book months in advance and must get here under their own power.

The trail ends at Mt. Tamalpais State Park's East Peak Visitor Center. From here, you can see parts of nine counties on clear days, including the majestic Sierra Nevada. In addition to the visitor center, there is a snack bar, restrooms, parking, and access to a number of hiking trails, including a 0.3-mile plank walk to the lookout tower at the top of the peak.

CONTACT marinwater.org/recreation and rtc.li/mount-tamalpais-sp

---

PARKING

Parking areas are located in Mill Valley and are listed from south to north. *Indicates that at least one accessible parking space is available.*

FERN CANYON ROAD On-street parking at end of Fern Canyon Road, 0.6 mile west of Summit Ave. (37.9208, -122.5675).

EAST PEAK VISITOR CENTER* End of E. Ridgecrest Blvd., 6.8 miles east of Fairfax-Bolinas Road (37.9273, -122.5801).

This history-filled trail traverses the communities of Upland, Rancho Cucamonga, Fontana, and Rialto in Southern California's Inland Empire metropolitan region. It follows the route of the Pacific Electric Railway, once the largest interurban railway on earth. The railway's San Bernardino Line, designed around the citrus industry, was completed in 1914.

The rail-trail is open to cyclists, walkers, runners, and equestrians and weaves its way through residential neighborhoods. Be prepared for on-street crossings that, while remarkably well-designed and marked, will add some time to your journey. There are no gaps along this 20-mile trail, so getting lost is not a concern. While some segments are rather utilitarian, others are tree lined, featuring charming plantings and landscaping, especially at crossings— look for the purple blooms of the jacaranda trees in the spring. You may catch a glimpse of mountain views on the

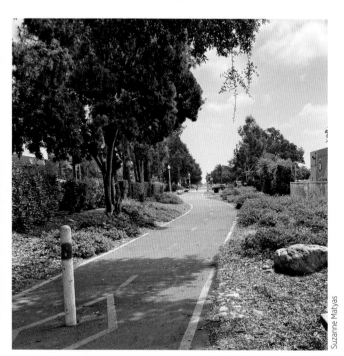

Connecting Claremont and Rialto, the rail-trail follows the old Pacific Electric Railway.

Counties
San Bernardino

Endpoints
Claremont Blvd. and Huntington Dr. (Upland); N. Cactus Ave., between W. Second St. and W. First St. (Rialto)

Mileage
20

Type
Rail-Trail

Roughness Rating
1

Surface
Asphalt, Concrete, Crushed Stone

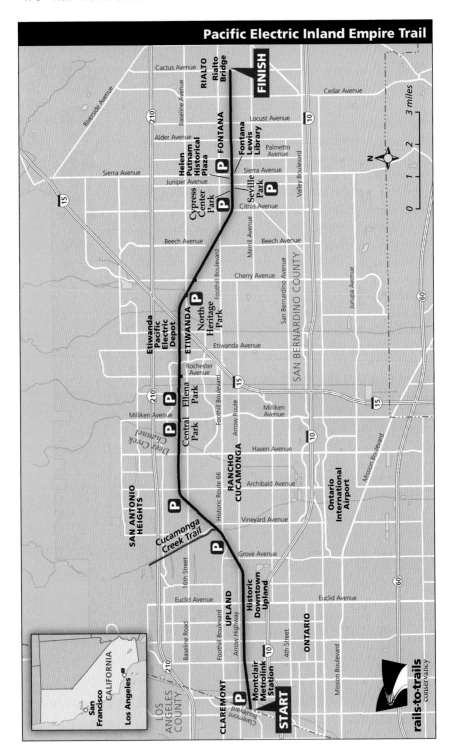

Pacific Electric Inland Empire Trail

Cactus Avenue

RIALTO

Rialto Bridge

FINISH

Riverside Avenue

Baseline Avenue

Cedar Avenue

210

Locust Avenue

10

Alder Avenue

FONTANA

Fontana Lewis Library

Palmetto Avenue

Sierra Avenue

Helen Putnam Historical Plaza

Sierra Avenue

Juniper Avenue

Seville Park

Valley Boulevard

Cypress Center Park

Citrus Avenue

15

Beech Avenue

Merrill Avenue

Beech Avenue

Cherry Avenue

San Bernardino Avenue

Jurupa Avenue

60

Etiwanda Pacific Electric Depot

ETIWANDA

North Heritage Park

SAN BERNARDINO COUNTY

Etiwanda Avenue

Rochester Avenue

Foothill Boulevard

15

15

210

Ellena Park

Foothill Boulevard

Arrow Route

Milliken Avenue

Milliken Avenue

10

Central Park

Deer Creek Channel

RANCHO CUCAMONGA

Haven Avenue

Historic Route 66

Archibald Avenue

Ontario International Airport

Mission Boulevard

SAN ANTONIO HEIGHTS

Vineyard Avenue

Cucamonga Creek Trail

16th Street

Grove Avenue

60

Euclid Avenue

UPLAND

Historic Downtown Upland

Euclid Avenue

Baseline Road

Foothill Boulevard

Arrow Highway

ONTARIO

4th Street

Mission Boulevard

210

Montclair Metrolink Station

10

CLAREMONT

Claremont Boulevard

START

LOS ANGELES COUNTY

N

0 1 2 3 miles

CALIFORNIA

San Francisco

Los Angeles

rails-to-trails conservancy

horizon, as well as small sculptures and a mural celebrating the corridor's railroad roots.

The Claremont and Montclair Metrolink stations are close to the start of the trail, providing a direct connection to Los Angeles's Union Station. Begin your journey at a trailhead at North Claremont Boulevard and Huntington Drive in Upland, just a few blocks from Pomona College. The first trail segment is on a slight hill. Once you cross Euclid Avenue, you will reach Historic Downtown Upland, where you can enjoy popular restaurants, do some shopping, or swing by the Saturday farmers market. Continuing, you will find small plazas with tables, benches, and chessboards at North 8th and North 10th Avenues. A half mile after crossing over Historic Route 66, you will intersect the paved, 2.4-mile Cucamonga Creek Trail. Farther north, past Haven Avenue, the Deer Creek Channel includes a trail that can be accessed here. Just before Milliken Avenue is a fitness court and the impeccably manicured Central Park, followed by Ellena Park at the next intersection.

You will leave the trail via buffered bike lanes at Rochester Avenue. At Etiwanda Avenue, take note of the Etiwanda Pacific Electric Depot, which served passengers until 1941 and freight until 1960. Between Oleander and Cypress Avenues is Cypress Center Park, situated next to Seville Park and Amphitheater. Past Juniper Avenue is the Helen Putnam Historical Plaza, which houses rose gardens and an old-fashioned windmill. You also will find the Art Depot, which served its original purpose as an agricultural freight depot from 1915 to 1961 and now holds classes, exhibits, and programming. Across from the gallery is the last parking area for this trail (there is no parking near the trail's eastern endpoint in Rialto).

On the next block, enjoy the fountains at the Fontana Lewis Library before passing yet another park. At Mango Avenue is the Fontana Citrus Association building (later renamed the Sunkist Packing Plant, it now functions as a warehouse for the Fontana Unified School District). The trail's grand finale is a bridge that replicates Venice, Italy's Rialto Bridge, for which the California city is allegedly named.

CONTACT petrail.weebly.com/map.html

continued on next page

PARKING

Parking areas are listed from west to east. *Indicates that at least one accessible parking space is available.*

UPLAND* Huntington Dr., off Claremont Blvd. (34.0952, -117.7036).

RANCHO CUCAMONGA* Foothill Blvd./Historic Rte. 66, between Baker Ave. and Highridge Pl. (34.1056, -117.6182).

RANCHO CUCAMONGA* Amethyst Ave., 200 feet south of Lomita Dr. (34.1237, -117.5984).

RANCHO CUCAMONGA* Central Park, at Milliken Ave. and Central Park (34.1236, -117.5596).

RANCHO CUCAMONGA* Ellena Park, Kenyon Way, between Ellena Dr. and Tortona Dr. (34.1247, -117.5503).

FONTANA* North end of North Heritage Park, N. Heritage Cir., 450 feet north of Del Norte St. (34.1244, -117.5041).

FONTANA* Cypress Center Park, Oleander and Seville Aves. (34.1015, -117.4488).

FONTANA* Seville Park and Amphitheater, Cypress and Seville Aves. (34.1015, -117.4439) and Seville and Juniper Aves. (34.1015, -117.4409).

FONTANA* Street parking on Seville Ave., between Bennett and Nuevo Aves. (34.1013, -117.4380).

The Richmond Greenway is a prime example of how activism and local champions can create a vibrant and well-used community asset. After sitting unused for more than a quarter century, a former rail line was transformed into a pathway through the heart of Richmond, an area that has been traditionally underserved with little green space.

The Richmond Greenway has brought with it community gardens, parks, richly colored murals, and green spaces all along its route while connecting neighbors to a larger regional trail network. The trail is part of a developing 2,600-miles-plus Bay Area regional trail network being spearheaded by the Bay Area Trails Collaborative (**railstotrails.org/bay-area**) and Rails-to-Trails Conservancy as a TrailNation™ project to increase safe walking, biking, and trail access for millions of Bay Area residents.

The western end of the trail is located where Ohio Avenue intersects Canal Boulevard/Richmond Parkway and continues as a well-marked two-way cycle track along

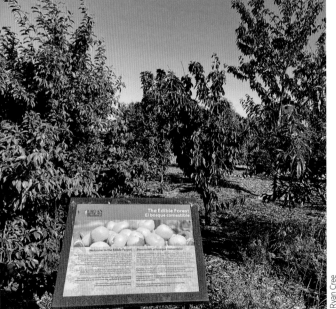

Ryan Cree

The 6th Street Community Garden brings an edible oasis to a dense urban area.

County
Contra Costa

Endpoints
W. Ohio Ave. and
Richmond Pkwy./Canal
Blvd. (Richmond);
San Pablo Ave., 0.1 mile
south of Macdonald Ave.
(El Cerrito)

Mileage
2.5

Type
Rail-Trail/Rail-with-Trail

Roughness Rating
1

Surface
Asphalt

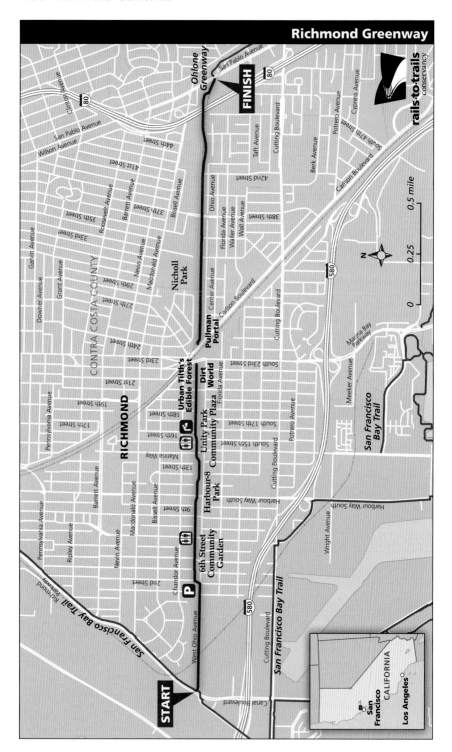

the north side of Ohio Avenue. At Second Street, the trail shifts to the former rail corridor through a parking lot with accessible spaces.

Between Fourth and Sixth Streets, the 6th Street Community Garden, operated by the nonprofit Urban Tilth, brings a green and edible oasis to an area with dense housing. Labeled garden plots, raised beds, and trellises—including the Berryland section, offering more than 18 varieties of edible berries—give the community a delicious and healthy selection of fresh produce to enjoy.

Between Eighth Street and Harbour Way, the trail traverses Harbour-8 Park, with vibrant murals, artwork, and play areas. Here, the Yellow Brick Road pathway provides a safe connection to the surrounding Iron Triangle community. Both the park and the pathway are projects of the nonprofit Pogo Park, whose mission is to transform derelict and little-used parks into safe, green, beautiful public spaces where children can play.

In 0.2 mile, just after crossing Marina Way, you'll reach Unity Park Community Plaza, a large public playground and green space. Take a stroll through Urban Tilth's Edible Forest of apple, plum, and other fruit-bearing trees. Trailside restrooms and water are available here. Just past the plaza is Dirt World, a pump track to test your off-road bike skills.

When you exit Dirt World, you'll arrive at 23rd Street, where there is a gap between the eastern and western portions of the trail. Although the gap is small, it is challenging to safely reach the next section; the on-road route to reach the eastern portion of the trail is not recommended for novice or insecure bikers. Clear wayfinding signage is planned but was not yet present as of the publication of this guidebook. Turn right on 23rd Street and travel south 0.4 mile on the bike lane. Take a left on Cutting Boulevard and, in 0.5 mile, take another left onto Carlson Boulevard (after crossing the railroad tracks); use caution as these streets do not have bike lanes. In 0.6 mile, you'll see an entrance for the trail on your right shortly after passing Ohio Avenue. Here, you'll find Pullman Portal, a small park that features a colorful mural celebrating Richmond's frontline workers.

The trail continues east as a rail-with-trail paralleling active commuter-rail lines (fenced off from the trail). There are multiple access points from local neighborhood streets, some with small community plots with murals and budding greenery. At 33rd Street, 0.4 mile east of Pullman Portal, a pedestrian bridge over the rail lines leads to Nicholl Park, which offers baseball diamonds, playgrounds, and a skate park. The trail continues 0.7 mile east to a tunnel under I-80. On the other side, the trail ends at San Pablo Avenue, where it meets up with the Ohlone Greenway (see page 161).

CONTACT richmondgreenway.org

continued on next page

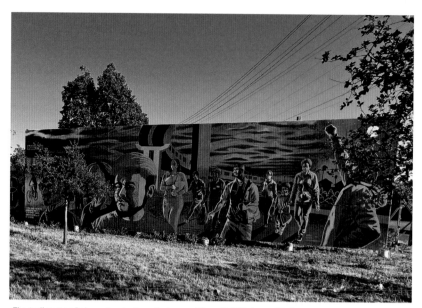

The trail passes Rebeca Garcia-González's mural Essential Workers of Pullman.   Joe LaCroix

---

PARKING

In addition to the parking area below, there are several opportunities along the route for on-street parking. *Indicates that at least one accessible parking space is available.*

RICHMOND* Second St., 145 feet north of Ohio Ave. (37.9313, -122.3678).

The Richmond–San Rafael Bridge Path provides safe passage between its two namesake communities located in Contra Costa and Marin Counties. At first glance, the pathway may seem more utilitarian than thrilling, but that's before you truly experience the bridge: pedaling along an interstate highway some 185 feet above the San Francisco Bay at its highest point is an adventure not soon forgotten.

The trail is also part of a developing 2,600-miles-plus Bay Area regional trail network being spearheaded by the Bay Area Trails Collaborative (**railstotrails.org/bay-area**) and Rails-to-Trails Conservancy as a TrailNation™ project to increase safe walking, biking, and trail access for millions of Bay Area residents.

The bridge itself first opened for service in 1956, but it wasn't until 2019—after decades of advocacy for safe accommodation—that it was opened to bicycle and pedestrian traffic. The bridge has stacked lanes traveling in each direction across the bay; the Richmond–San Rafael

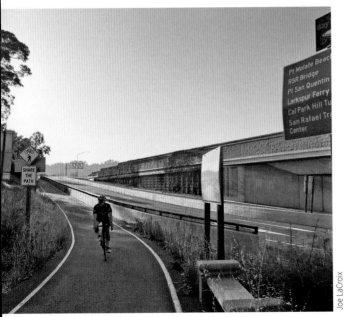

Joe LaCroix

The Richmond–San Rafael Bridge Path connects its two namesake communities in Contra Costa and Marin counties.

Counties
Contra Costa, Marin

Endpoints
Point San Quentin at Jean & John Starkweather Shoreline Park (San Rafael); Castro St. and Tewksbury Ave. (Richmond)

Mileage
6

Type
Greenway/Non-Rail-Trail

Roughness Rating
1

Surface
Asphalt, Concrete

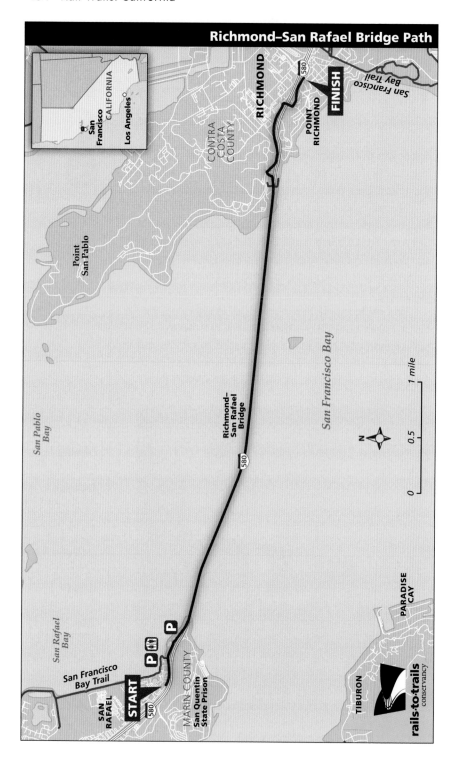

Bridge Path shares the upper deck with westbound automobiles, though it's well separated from traffic by concrete barriers.

Starting at the western end in San Rafael's Jean & John Starkweather Shoreline Park, you'll have access to restrooms, parking, and the San Francisco Bay Trail, a planned 500-mile pathway encircling the bay and connecting more than 130 parks. Exit the park to the west, traveling through a large parking area, and pop out onto Francisco Boulevard East. Turn left and ride east on-road or on the sidewalk 0.3 mile to a small trailhead facility (the entrance will be on your left) at Francisco Boulevard East and Main Street for expansive views of the bay.

Continuing east, the height and enormity of the double-decker bridge start to build as you approach it. Be prepared for a modest climb but consummate rewards when you reach the top of the bridge's arc: unobstructed views of the San Francisco Bay to the north and, weather permitting, glimpses of San Francisco to the south.

At the eastern end of the bridge, the path continues another 1.5 miles to its endpoint at the intersection of Castro Street and Tewksbury Avenue. A bollard-separated bike lane provides additional access along the lightly trafficked Tewksbury Avenue into the quaint Point Richmond neighborhood, which is full of great eating and entertainment options. Take some time to explore. There is a bike-share station on Tewksbury Avenue at the Castro Street pathway entrance.

CONTACT rtc.li/mtc-ca

PARKING

Parking areas are located within San Rafael and are listed from west to east. *Indicates that at least one accessible parking space is available.*

JEAN & JOHN STARKWEATHER SHORELINE PARK* Accessible from Francisco Blvd. E., 0.3 mile east of Morphew St. Look for a small blue sign labeled **Public Shore Parking** directing you into a parking lot for the Bay Park Center; drive through this private lot to a dead end where parking for the park is located (37.9455, -122.4838).

POINT SAN QUENTIN PARKING* Francisco Blvd. E. and Main St. (37.9440, -122.4802); parking is limited.

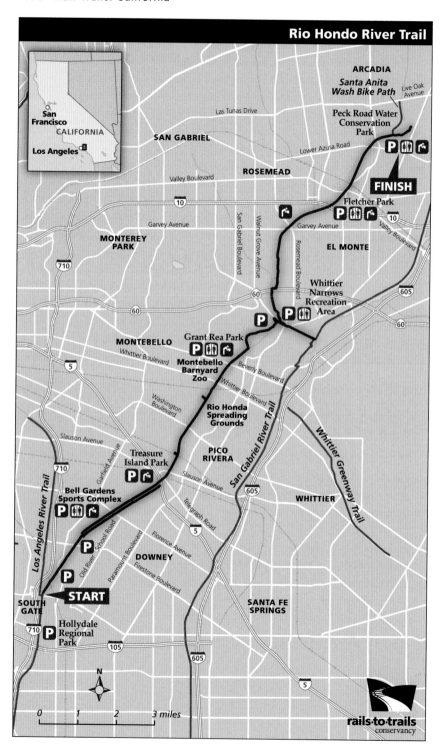

Rio Hondo River Trail

ARCADIA

Santa Anita Wash Bike Path

Live Oak Avenue

Peck Road Water Conservation Park

Las Tunas Drive

SAN GABRIEL

Lower Azusa Road

ROSEMEAD

FINISH

Valley Boulevard

Fletcher Park

10

Garvey Avenue

EL MONTE

MONTEREY PARK

Garvey Avenue

710

San Gabriel Boulevard

Walnut Grove Avenue

60

Rosemead Boulevard

Whittier Narrows Recreation Area

605

60

Grant Rea Park

MONTEBELLO

Whittier Boulevard

Montebello Barnyard Zoo

Beverly Boulevard

Whittier Boulevard

San Gabriel River Trail

5

Washington Boulevard

Rio Honda Spreading Grounds

Whittier Greenway Trail

Slauson Avenue

Treasure Island Park

PICO RIVERA

WHITTIER

710

Garfield Avenue

Bell Gardens Sports Complex

Slauson Avenue

605

Los Angeles River Trail

Old River School Road

Telegraph Road

5

P

Florence Avenue

Paramount Boulevard

DOWNEY

Firestone Boulevard

SANTA FE SPRINGS

P

START

SOUTH GATE

710

Hollydale Regional Park

105

605

5

N

0   1   2   3 miles

San Francisco

CALIFORNIA

Los Angeles

The emerging trail system in and around the greater Los Angeles area may surprise visitors. The 17-mile Rio Hondo River Trail has become a key component of this system. While much of it follows the concrete drainage channel for Rio Hondo through urban and suburban sprawl, two sections follow the river on open ground with varied landscapes.

The trail starts where the Rio Hondo (Spanish for "deep river") meets the Los Angeles River and the Los Angeles River Greenway, which heads south 12 miles to the Port of Long Beach. While there's an entrance ramp to the Rio Hondo Trail on the east side of the river on Imperial Highway in Lynwood, the trailhead closest to parking is 1.5 miles south in Hollydale Regional Park in South Gate.

As you make your way along the channel, you're often traveling below the surrounding terrain without noticing whether you're in residential, commercial, or industrial districts. An advantage is you don't have to stop for the cross streets that pass overhead. In addition, the trail runs

County
Los Angeles

Endpoints
Los Angeles River Trail
at Imperial Hwy.,
0.3 mile west of Garfield
Pl. (South Gate);
Live Oak Ave., between
Hempstead Ave. and
Eighth Ave. (Arcadia)

Mileage
17.8

Type
Greenway/Non-Rail-Trail

Roughness Rating
1

Surface
Asphalt, Concrete

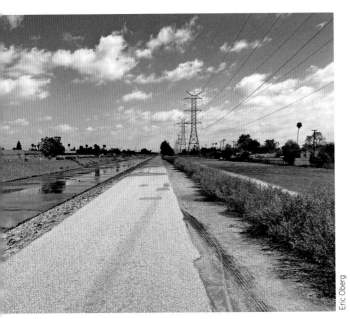

Eric Oberg

Much of the trail follows the concrete drainage channel for the Rio Hondo through urban and suburban areas.

on both sides of the channel in one 3-mile segment, making it more accessible to local residents.

About 4.7 miles along the route, you'll notice a natural landscape along the corridor in what is called the Rio Hondo Spreading Grounds. This is a 2-mile stretch where water is allowed to leave the concrete channel and percolate into the soil. Heading north, keep a keen eye out for the Montebello Barnyard Zoo on the north side of the trail. It's not unusual to look up and find an ostrich or a donkey checking out the happenings on the trail.

About 2 miles north of the spreading grounds, you'll take a switchback up the side of a dam structure and enter the 1,500-acre Whittier Narrows Recreation Area. The scenery changes dramatically from concrete channel to wide-open wetland sanctuary with woodlands typical of river shorelines and lakes. You might see migrating waterfowl in season in the 400-acre Whittier Narrows Natural Area. Crossing San Gabriel Boulevard, you'll continue north along the natural drainage 3.3 miles before reentering the concrete channel. At 0.3 mile east of the San Gabriel Boulevard crossing, you could take a connector trail 1.2 miles east to the San Gabriel River Trail (see page 211).

Continuing in the concrete channel, you'll pass Fletcher Park and notice that an elevated railway accompanies the trail through the city of El Monte.

An elevated railway runs alongside the trail through the city of El Monte.   Eric Oberg

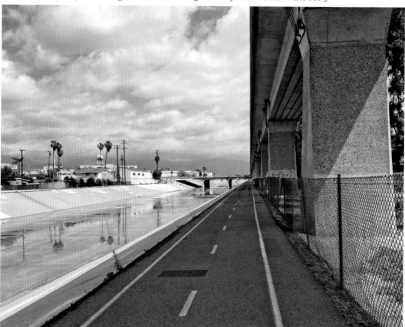

Climbing the dam to a reservoir about a mile past the San Gabriel Valley Airport, take the right fork (a left takes you onto the Santa Anita Wash Bike Path) and continue 0.6 mile to the Peck Road Water Conservation Park, where you'll find parking, restrooms, drinking water, and shaded picnic tables.

CONTACT rtc.li/rio-hondo-river-trail

PARKING

Parking areas are listed from south to north. *Indicates that at least one accessible parking space is available.*

SOUTH GATE* Hollydale Regional Park, 5400 Monroe Ave. at Los Angeles River Trail (33.9221, -118.1757).

SOUTH GATE* Circle Park, 10129 Garfield Ave. (33.9384, -118.1680).

DOWNEY* Rio Hondo Dr. and Dinwiddie St. (33.9528, -118.1565).

BELL GARDENS* Sports Complex, 8000 Park Lane (33.9588, -118.1539).

DOWNEY* Treasure Island Park, 9300 S. Bluff Road (33.9663, -118.1341).

MONTEBELLO* Grant Rea Park, 600 Rea Dr. (34.0164, -118.0915).

MONTEBELLO* Whittier Narrows Reservoir, 989 Lincoln Ave. (34.0241, -118.0851).

SOUTH EL MONTE* Bosque del Rio Hondo, 9311 San Gabriel Blvd. (34.0292, -118.0682).

EL MONTE* Fletcher Park, 3404 Fletcher Park Way (34.0710, -118.0481).

ARCADIA* Peck Road Water Conservation Park, 5401 Peck Road (34.1000, -118.0117).

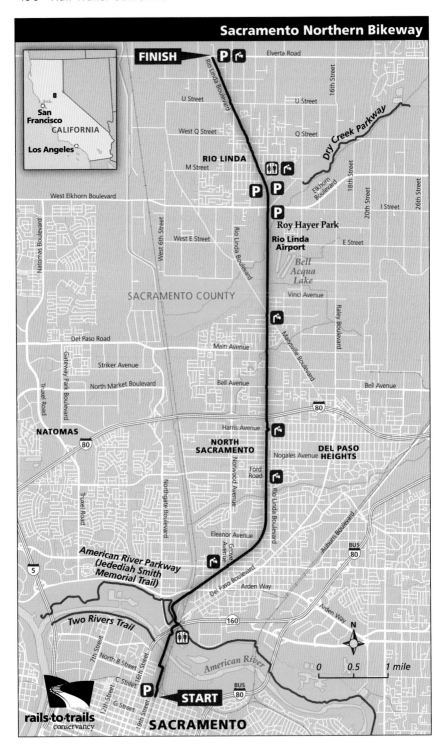

Sacramento Northern Bikeway

The Sacramento Northern Bikeway gives visitors a taste of California's capital city as it crosses the fabled American River and passes into the once prosperous suburbs of North Sacramento. Adopted as a commuter route by many downtown workers, the 10-mile paved trail takes a mostly straight, flat route that connects residential and commercial areas with parks offering welcome relief from the summer sun. It ends in an agricultural area in the north.

The trail follows the former 93-mile right-of-way opened by the Chico Electric Railway between Chico and Sacramento in 1904. Operating under several entities, it eventually became the Sacramento Northern Railway in 1925, with interurban service from Chico to San Francisco. Passenger service ended in 1941, although the railway carried freight into the 1970s.

The trail starts at the Sacramento Northern Bikeway arch on C Street, just 200 feet east of 19th Street, in the Blue Diamond Almonds headquarters district. On-street

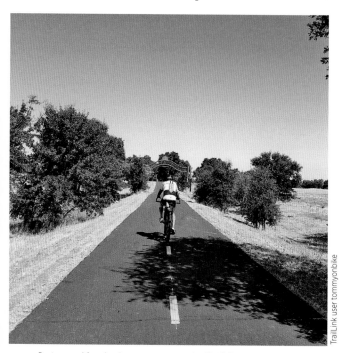

Pasture and farmland emerge as you enter North Sacramento.

County
Sacramento

Endpoints
C St., 200 feet east of 19th St. (Sacramento);
Rio Linda Blvd. and Elverta Road (Elverta)

Mileage
10.1

Type
Rail-Trail

Roughness Rating
1

Surface
Asphalt

parking is available here and along much of the trail, which is accessible at frequent street intersections along its length.

You might encounter encampments of unhoused people in the trail corridor along the southern 2 or 3 miles. Bicyclists passing through these areas should watch out for dogs and pedestrians crossing the trail.

Shortly after departing the arch, the trail intersects the developing Two Rivers Trail, which begins in Tiscornia Park to the west and will extend to H Street when complete. The bikeway then crosses the American River on a 600-foot bridge left over from the railroad days. Stay on the paved trail as it curves under highway overpasses, and turn left onto the American River Parkway (see page 13) at a T intersection. In 100 yards, take the right fork back onto the Sacramento Northern Bikeway.

You'll soon leave the greenway along the river and enter the former city of North Sacramento. Founded in 1924, it thrived as a bedroom community with its own business district. The opening of a bypass hurt merchants in the 1950s, and the City of Sacramento annexed the town in the 1960s.

Occasional groves of trees offer shade along the exposed bike path. Look for trailside kiosks that offer mini oases at Grove Avenue, Ford Road, Harris Avenue, and Marysville Boulevard.

Pasture and farmland emerge as you leave Sacramento after about 6 miles. The Rio Linda Airport is on your right, just after three ponds of the Bell Acqua Lake water-skiing site. Passing the airport, you might hear the whining engines of midget cars racing at Roy Hayer Park or the whinnying of horses at the Central Park Horse Arena; horse riding is allowed on the trail north of Sacramento, in Rio Linda.

In about 0.6 mile, you'll come to the Rio Linda park district headquarters, which has a playground and shade. A half block farther, you'll find a replica of the original Rio Linda rail depot, which houses the Rio Linda Chamber of Commerce. The trail ends in 2 miles at Elverta Road.

CONTACT rtc.li/sacramento-co-parks

PARKING

Parking areas are listed from south to north. *Indicates that at least one accessible parking space is available.*

SACRAMENTO C St. and 19th St. (38.5847, -121.4776); on-street parking.

RIO LINDA* Cherry Lane, 300 feet south of Elkhorn Blvd. (38.6829, -121.4466).

RIO LINDA* Recreation and Park District, 810 Oak Lane (38.6887, -121.4481).

RIO LINDA* Chamber of Commerce, 6730 Front St. (38.6904, -121.4493).

ELVERTA* Park and ride, 7945 Rio Linda Blvd. (38.7139, -121.4627).

In the 19th century, thousands of Forty-Niners passed through Sacramento on their way to California's gold fields. Today, visitors can explore those former haunts in the Old Sacramento Waterfront District from the Sacramento River Parkway Trail.

The 9.3-mile trail hugs the levees on the eastern bank of the Sacramento River as it rolls south from that river's confluence with the American River. It links to both the American River Parkway (see page 13) and the Two Rivers Trail in the north. After a 2-mile interruption through the Pocket neighborhood, it resumes for about 3 miles to its endpoint at a sports complex in the Freeport neighborhood.

Development of the trail began in the mid-1970s. It's the northernmost segment of the Great California Delta Trail, which was envisioned as a corridor along the California Delta that will join the San Francisco Bay Trail system.

The paved trail starts at the base of the Jibboom Street bridge at Tiscornia Park, where the American River flows into the Sacramento. More parking and facilities are available across the bridge at Discovery Park.

County
Sacramento

Endpoints
Northern segment: Tiscornia Park at Jibboom St., 0.2 mile northwest of Richards Blvd. (Sacramento); Ellsworth C. Zacharias Park, Clipper Way, 0.1 mile east of Riverton Way (Sacramento) *Southern segment:* Garcia Bend Park at Pocket Road between Roberts River Way and Windbridge Dr. (Sacramento); Bill Conlin Sports Complex at Freeport Blvd., 0.5 mile north of Cosumnes River Blvd. (Sacramento)

Mileage
9.3

Type
Rail-Trail

Roughness Rating
1

Surface
Asphalt, Concrete

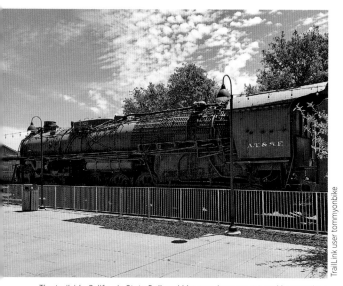

The trailside California State Railroad Museum houses restored locomotives and a historic depot.

TrailLink user tommyonbike

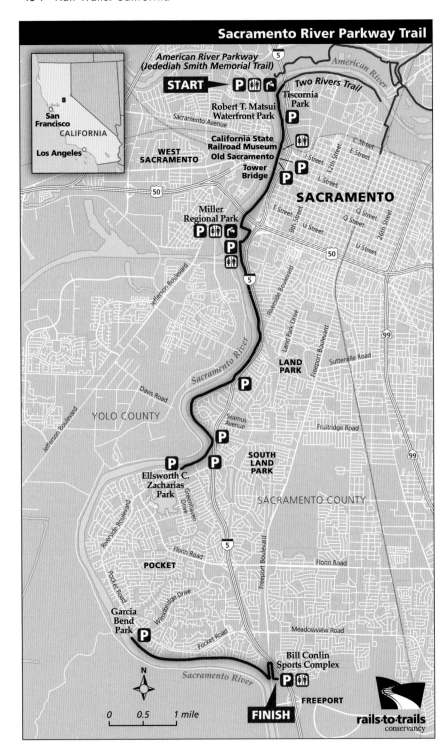

Sacramento River Parkway Trail

American River Parkway
(Jedediah Smith Memorial Trail)

5

American River

START

Two Rivers Trail

Tiscornia Park

Robert T. Matsui
Waterfront Park

Sacramento Avenue

California State
Railroad Museum
Old Sacramento

Tower
Bridge

WEST
SACRAMENTO

C Street
E Street

I Street

12th Street

L Street

SACRAMENTO

50

Miller
Regional Park

T Street

9th Street

T Street

U Street

Q Street
Q Street

26th Street

U Street

5

Jefferson Boulevard

Sacramento River

Riverside Boulevard

50

U Street

99

LAND
PARK

Land Park Drive

Freeport Boulevard

Sutterville Road

Davis Road

YOLO COUNTY

Seamus
Avenue

Fruitridge Road

SOUTH
LAND
PARK

99

Ellsworth C.
Zacharias
Park

Greenhaven Drive

SACRAMENTO COUNTY

Riverside Boulevard

POCKET

Florin Road

5

Windbridge Drive

Freeport Boulevard

Florin Road

Pocket Road

Garcia
Bend
Park

Pocket Road

Meadowview Road

Bill Conlin
Sports Complex

N

Sacramento River

0   0.5   1 mile

FINISH

FREEPORT

rails·to·trails
conservancy

San
Francisco

CALIFORNIA

Los Angeles

Heading south for about a mile atop a levee built to protect Sacramento from flooding, you'll arrive at the old railyards, once the largest in the west. The vintage rolling stock here indicates your arrival in Old Sacramento. Here, you'll find the California State Railroad Museum, which houses many restored locomotives and cars, as well as a historic depot. Nearby, you can take a short excursion on the Sacramento Southern Railroad, a tourist train that once carried freight and passengers in the early 20th century.

The parkway's river walk through Old Sacramento can get crowded with tourists hopping in and out of shops, restaurants, and bars. An alternative is Front Street, which is wider but paved with cobblestones and just as busy. The trail gets more manageable after you pass Capitol Mall/CA 275 at the iconic Tower Bridge.

South of the bridge, the trail is wedged between the excursion train tracks and the river. About 1.5 miles past the Tower Bridge, you'll pass a marina and launch ramp in shady Miller Regional Park.

There are more parks along the trail for the next 4 miles to the community of Pocket, named for the semicircular bend in the river. Access to the levee is broken here, but plans are underway to upgrade the levee to a trail after property is acquired. Until that happens, take Clipper Way south to Riverside Boulevard, and turn right to continue on Riverside (it becomes Pocket Road) about 3.7 miles to Garcia Bend Park to rejoin the trail. You'll reach the end of the trail in 3 miles at the Bill Conlin Sports Complex in Freeport.

Unless you're familiar with the area, check the U.S. Army Corps of Engineers website (**rtc.li/sacramento-river-levees**) before you go for possible levee closings due to construction.

CONTACT rtc.li/sacramento-bikeways

continued on next page

PARKING

Parking areas are located within Sacramento and are listed from north to south. Select parking areas for the trail are listed below. For a detailed list of parking areas and other waypoints, go to **TrailLink.com**™. *Indicates that at least one accessible parking space is available.*

TISCORNIA PARK* 195 Jibboom St. (38.5977, -121.5064). If you're traveling on Jibboom St. from the north, you'll turn left across from the trail to exit into the parking lot. If you are traveling from the south, you'll turn right into the exit.

ROBERT T. MATSUI WATERFRONT PARK* Jibboom St., 0.2 mile north of Railyards Blvd. (38.5917, -121.5052).

MILLER REGIONAL PARK* Marina View Dr., beginning 200 feet south of Broadway (38.5672, -121.5185); paid parking.

MILLER REGIONAL PARK* 2706 Ramp Way (38.5648, -121.5164).

CAPTAINS TABLE ROAD* 1000 Captains Table Road, 0.2 mile north of Riverside Blvd. (38.5360, -121.5163).

RIVERSIDE BLVD. Between Rio Viale Ct. and 35th Ave. (38.5199, -121.5230).

GARCIA BEND PARK* 7654 Pocket Road, between Roberts River Way and Windbridge Dr. (38.4790, -121.5430).

BILL CONLIN SPORTS COMPLEX* 7895 Freeport Blvd. (38.4708, -121.5027).

On-street, metered parking can be found on Front St. between L St. and J St. (38.5834, -121.5054).

The northern endpoint of the Sacramento River Rail Trail offers views of the country's eighth-largest dam and California's largest reservoir—Shasta Lake—and the often snowcapped Mount Shasta. Before you jump on the trail, explore the Shasta Dam Visitor Center, which is run by the U.S. Department of the Interior. Learn about the area's history, grab a brochure on Redding trails, or enjoy a picnic amid the mountain scenery. You might even see wildlife, such as deer and osprey. Built during the Great Depression and throughout World War II, the 602-foot dam was considered an engineering marvel, and today it helps water one of the world's leading agricultural producers: California's Central Valley.

To start your trail adventure, head to the Shasta Dam Trailhead, where parking and restrooms are available. For the first 8 miles heading south, the trail leisurely follows the Sacramento River, which feeds off Shasta Lake. Shady nooks lined with ponderosa pines punctuate the peaceful route, and a 500-foot former rail tunnel adds to the

County
Shasta

Endpoints
Shasta Dam Trailhead, 2.8 miles south of Shasta Dam Visitor Center (Redding); Keswick Trailhead, West St./Rock Creek Road and Iron Mountain Road (Redding); FB Trailhead, Keswick Dam Road, 0.4 mile south of Keswick Dam (Redding)

Mileage
11.1

Type
Rail-Trail

Roughness Rating
1–2

Surface
Asphalt

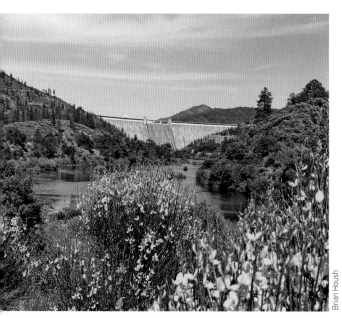

Brian Housh

The rail-trail's northern end offers vistas of Shasta Dam, the country's eighth-largest dam.

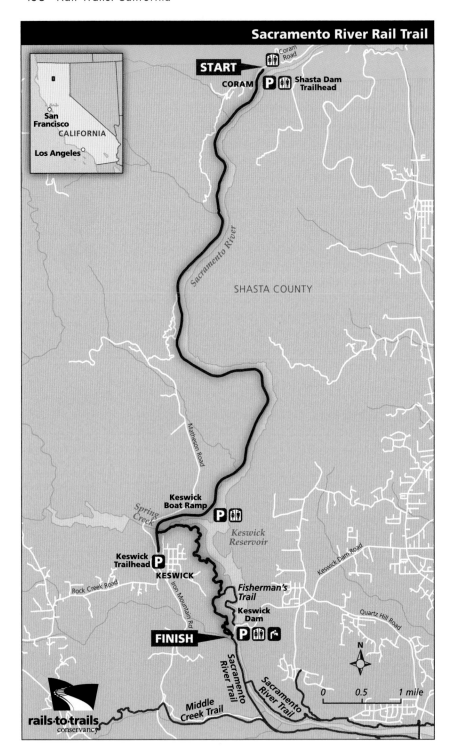

Sacramento River Rail Trail

CALIFORNIA

San Francisco

Los Angeles

START

CORAM

Shasta Dam Trailhead

Coram Road

Sacramento River

SHASTA COUNTY

Matheson Road

Keswick Boat Ramp

Spring Creek

Keswick Reservoir

Keswick Trailhead

KESWICK

Rock Creek Road

Iron Mountain Rd

Keswick Dam Road

Quartz Hill Road

Fisherman's Trail

Keswick Dam

FINISH

N

0   0.5   1 mile

Sacramento River Trail

Sacramento River Trail

Middle Creek Trail

rails·to·trails
conservancy

relaxing trek along the tranquil river. In the early 1900s, the railroad provided services to the copper mining town of Coram.

For a more meditative experience, you can either end your trip at the Keswick Boat Ramp (mile 7) or head south after crossing Spring Creek to reach the Keswick Trailhead (mile 8), one of the trail's two southern endpoints.

Alternatively, to raise your heartbeat, head east after crossing Spring Creek and continue 2.8 miles, where you'll travel a portion of the trail dubbed "the roller coaster" by locals for its cardio workout. Winding hills flank Keswick Reservoir, a stretch of the Sacramento River that leads to Keswick Dam, the other southern endpoint. Make sure you have plenty of water for these steep, staggered hills. Any rest breaks are rewarded with beautiful views of the blue-green water, rich-hued soil, lush vegetation, and mountains in the distance. A 2-mile path called the Fisherman's Trail shoots off from this part of the Sacramento River Rail Trail, leading to the reservoir with an access point from Keswick Dam Road. As its name suggests, the trail is used to access fishing at the reservoir as it skates along the banks leading up to the dam. Check the California Department of Fish and Wildlife's resources on fishing regulations in Shasta County at **wildlife.ca.gov/regions/1**. In the springtime, you can enjoy delightful wildflowers as you head to your fishing spot.

End your journey at a trailhead off Keswick Dam Road, where you can picnic at the top of a hill overlooking the dam. To continue your adventure, carefully cross the winding road to start the 12-mile Sacramento River Trail (see page 201), which leads you to the city of Redding and its picturesque Sundial Bridge.

CONTACT visitredding.com/get-outside/trails

PARKING

Parking areas are located within Redding and are listed from north to south. *Indicates that at least one accessible parking space is available.*

SHASTA DAM TRAILHEAD Gravel parking lot off Coram Road, 2.8 miles south of Shasta Dam Visitor Center (40.7112, -122.4408).

KESWICK BOAT RAMP* Keswick Lake Ramp Road, 0.3 mile southeast of Iron Mountain Road (40.6324, -122.4530).

KESWICK TRAILHEAD* West St./Rock Creek Road and Iron Mountain Road (40.6247, -122.4660).

FB TRAILHEAD* Keswick Dam Road, 0.9 mile southeast of Iron Mountain Road (40.6100, -122.4481).

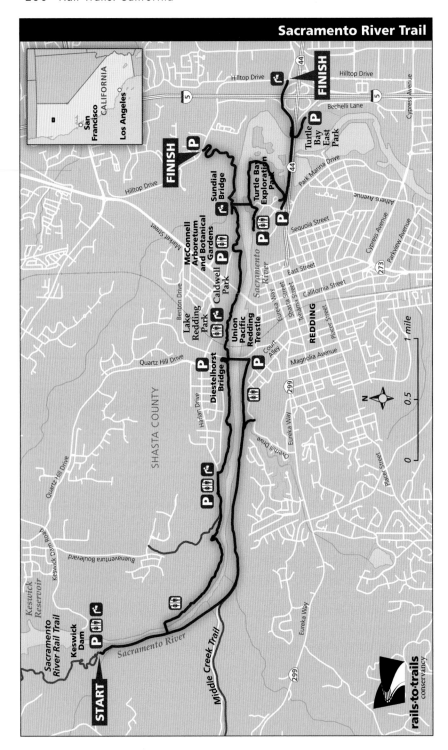

Sacramento River Trail

CALIFORNIA

San Francisco

Los Angeles

Hilltop Drive

FINISH

Hilltop Drive

Bechelli Lane

Cypress Avenue

Turtle Bay East Park

Park Marina Drive

Athens Avenue

FINISH

P

Hilltop Drive

Sundial Bridge

Turtle Bay Exploration Park

Sequoia Street

Cypress Avenue

Parkview Avenue

273

Market Street

McConnell Arboretum and Botanical Gardens

Sacramento River

East Street

Eureka Way

California Street

Shasta Street

Tehama Street

Placer Street

Caldwell Park

Benton Drive

Lake Redding Park

Union Pacific Redding Trestle

REDDING

Quartz Hill Drive

Diestelhorst Bridge

Court Alley

Magnolia Avenue

299

SHASTA COUNTY

Harlan Drive

Eureka Way

N

1 mile

0.5

0

Quartz Hill Drive

Buenaventura Boulevard

Overhill Drive

Eureka Way

Placer Street

Keswick Dam Road

Keswick Reservoir

Sacramento River Rail Trail

Keswick Dam

P

START

Sacramento River

Middle Creek Trail

299

rails-to-trails conservancy

For fans of loop trails, Northern California's Sacramento River Trail offers a diversity of options to avoid backtracking and to discover new places. This 12.3-mile paved trail provides an east–west route across central Redding, running through urban, suburban, and natural areas—all along the river.

The western endpoint offers a connection with the similarly named Sacramento River Rail Trail (see page 197), an 11.1-mile route up to the massive Shasta Dam. At the juncture of the two trails, alongside the more modest Keswick Dam, is a parking lot and trailhead. Heading south from the trailhead, the Sacramento River Trail splits after 0.6 mile to run on both sides of the river, enabling you to make it a loop. To reach the north side of the river, you cross a charming bicycle and pedestrian bridge designed to look like an old "swinging" bridge.

County
Shasta

Endpoints
Keswick Dam Road, 0.9 mile southeast of Iron Mountain Road (Redding); Aoki Way, 0.1 mile west of Sundial Bridge Dr. (Redding); Hilltop Dr., between St. Thomas Pkwy. and Sandpoint Dr. (Redding); dead end of Bechelli Lane at Turtle Bay East Park (Redding); Hilltop Dr. and Dana Dr. (Redding)

Mileage
12.3

Type
Rail-Trail

Roughness Rating
1

Surface
Asphalt

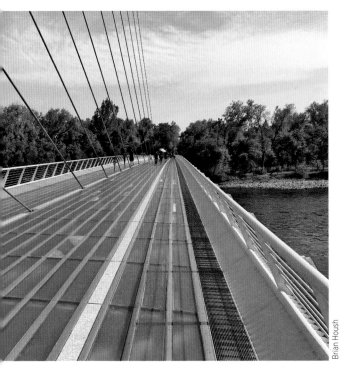

Brian Housh

The trail's centerpiece is the Sundial Bridge, designed by Spanish architect Santiago Calatrava.

In 2.6 miles, the trail enters central Redding and reaches the Diestelhorst Bridge, which you can cross to return to the south side of the river on your way back. Listed on the National Register of Historic Places, this bridge was built in 1915 and spans more than 600 feet. From it, rail fans will appreciate the view of the paralleling Union Pacific Redding Trestle, which soars 110 feet over the Sacramento River and remains active.

From the Diestelhorst Bridge, the trail continues east on the north side of the Sacramento River. At the base of the bridge, you'll enter Lake Redding Park and travel under the trestle as you enter the adjacent Caldwell Park. After 1.4 miles, you'll reach the centerpiece of the trail: the stunning, 700-foot-long Sundial Bridge, designed by Spanish architect Santiago Calatrava, whose works often evoke birds and wings. In its unique design, the towering mast of the cable-stayed bridge serves as the gnomon of a sundial, casting a shadow on a large dial in the adjoining park. You'll cross the bridge's glass-block walkway,

The towering mast of the Sundial Bridge serves as the gnomon of a massive sundial.   Brian Housh

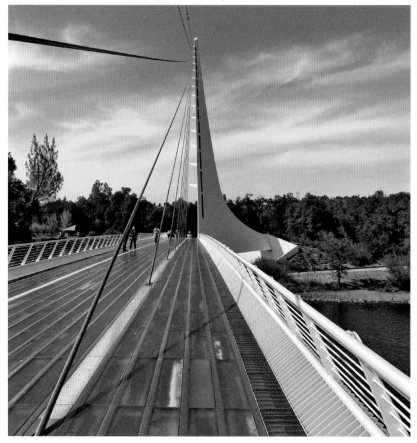

touching down in Turtle Bay Exploration Park on the south side of the river. As you travel through the park, you'll be sheltered by a lush tree canopy and can stop at the many benches along the river to enjoy the views. The 300-acre park also offers a museum, animal exhibits, playgrounds, and gardens.

On either side of the river, the trail continues a short distance to points east. On the south side of the river and south of Turtle Bay Exploration Park, the trail continues along CA 44 for 1 mile to Mt. Shasta Mall. On the north side of the river, the trail travels 0.9 mile to a residential neighborhood along Hilltop Drive.

CONTACT rtc.li/redding-parks

P A R K I N G

Parking areas are located within Redding and are listed from west to east. *Indicates that at least one accessible parking space is available.*

KESWICK DAM*: Keswick Dam Road, 0.9 mile southeast of Iron Mountain Road (40.6100, -122.4481).

HARLAN TRAILHEAD Dead end of Harlan Dr., 0.2 mile west of Lake Redding Dr. (40.5952, -122.4217).

DIESTELHORST BRIDGE (north side)* Benton Dr., 0.1 mile south of Quartz Hill Road (40.5949, -122.4023).

DIESTELHORST BRIDGE (south side)*: Middle Creek Road and Benton Dr. (40.5918, -122.4024).

MCCONNELL ARBORETUM AND BOTANICAL GARDENS 1500 Traveled Way (40.5932, -122.3851).

TURTLE BAY EXPLORATION PARK* 872–880 Sundial Bridge Dr. (40.5900, -122.3783).

TURTLE BAY EXPLORATION PARK* Sundial Bridge Dr., 0.2 mile north of Park Marina Dr. (40.5879, -122.3771).

TURTLE BAY EAST PARK* Dead end of Bechelli Lane, 1 mile north of Cypress Dr. (40.5842, -122.3638).

On-street parking is available on Hilltop Dr. between St. Thomas Pkwy. and Sandpoint Dr. (40.5973, -122.3692).

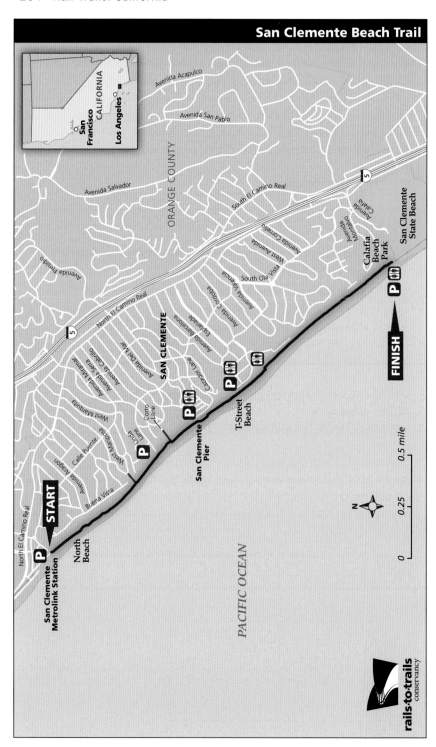

San Clemente Beach Trail

There's nothing like a day at the beach, especially in Southern California. The 2.3-mile San Clemente Beach Trail rolls between sandy bluffs and a wide-open beach at the edge of San Clemente, which calls itself The Spanish Village by the Sea. The rail-with-trail is a segment of the California Coastal Trail, a network of bicycling and hiking trails that, when complete, will stretch along the coastline for 1,230 miles from Oregon to the Mexican border.

The mostly packed-sand trail runs between the San Clemente Metrolink Station in the north and Calafia Beach Park in the south, near San Clemente State Beach. The trail shares a corridor with tracks used frequently by Amtrak and Metrolink commuter trains; cross the tracks only in designated areas. Also, bicyclists are required to walk their rides in other marked areas, specifically across bridges; the access points to the San Clemente Pier (located midway along the trail); and, during the summer,

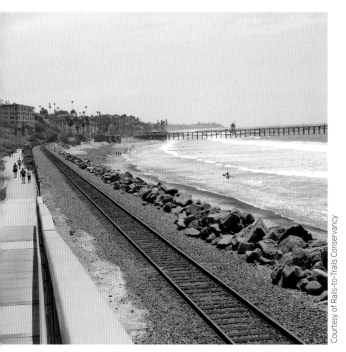

Courtesy of Rails-to-Trails Conservancy

The rail-with-trail rolls between sandy bluffs and a beach at the edge of San Clemente.

County
Orange

Endpoints
San Clemente Metrolink Station (San Clemente); Calafia Beach Park (San Clemente)

Mileage
2.3

Type
Rail-with-Trail

Roughness Rating
1–2

Surface
Boardwalk, Sand

a 0.2-mile stretch of trail from the pier south to Trafalgar Canyon Bridge. Bikes are not permitted on the pier, but bike parking is available at its base.

There are several places along the route to access the trail, but these are in neighborhoods up on the bluff and require using steep stairs. Level access for bicyclists and wheelchair users is available at the pier and at the northern and southern trailheads, which also have facilities and paid parking. Two sections of the trail are accessible for wheelchair users: the northern 0.6 mile, from North Beach south to West Mariposa, and a 0.3-mile central section, from Linda Lane to the pier.

Starting at North Beach near the Metrolink station, you'll find a small café with outdoor dining. Tall palm trees and whitewashed stucco buildings add to the coastal feel. Heading south, you'll come to a wooden walkway in 0.3 mile that runs along the base of a sandy bluff for 0.3 mile. Use the rail underpasses to get to the beaches.

The San Clemente Pier juts more than 1,000 feet into the Pacific Ocean about 1 mile south of North Beach. There's a restaurant at the base of the wooden pier, and you can walk out to the end to discuss the catch of the day with local anglers or watch surfers ride the waves. It's a short jaunt across the tracks to other shops and diners.

In 0.4 mile, the trail crosses back over to the east side of the tracks with an at-grade crossing just past T-Street Beach. It ends in another 0.9 mile at a parking lot for Calafia Beach Park, where you'll find another beachfront café.

San Clemente State Beach, offering more than a mile of beach, lies just beyond the end of the trail. You might find sea lions lolling along the shoreline, and small mammals, lizards, and snakes on the towering sandstone cliffs. Check the skies for coastal raptors as well as wild Amazon parrots.

CONTACT san-clemente.org/recreation-community/parks-trails/trails

PARKING

Parking areas are located within San Clemente and are listed from north to south. *Indicates that at least one accessible parking space is available.*

SAN CLEMENTE METROLINK STATION* Avenida Estacion and Calle Deshecha (33.4323, -117.6329).

LINDA LANE PARK* 340–398 Linda Lane (33.4232, -117.6226).

SAN CLEMENTE PIER* Avenida Victoria and Avenida Del Mar (33.4212, -117.6193).

T-STREET BEACH*: W. Paseo De Cristobal and Esplanade (33.4172, -117.6174).

CALAFIA BEACH PARK* End of Avenida Calafia, 0.3 mile southwest of Avenida Del Presidente (33.4057, -117.6066).

The San Diego Creek Trail is a spine of Irvine's extensive network of trails and bike lanes. Much of the trail follows San Diego Creek and connects to the city's well-appointed parks, schools, and residential subdivisions. Near its western endpoint in Newport Beach, the trail also runs adjacent to the Upper Newport Bay Nature Preserve, a protected estuary and renowned bird-watching area.

From end to end, the paved trail spans approximately 10 miles and provides a wide, well-maintained route for cyclists, walkers, and runners. Following the creek, it provides scenic views with cool, shaded areas near community and school park facilities. The city manages the trail as part of its nearly 400-mile (and still expanding) network of well-connected multiuse trails and on-street bicycle facilities, or bikeways. Many shorter bikeways touch or cross the San Diego Creek Trail at some point, allowing you to form loop trips. These include the University Trail,

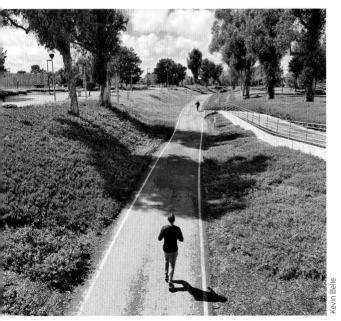

Beginning in Newport Beach, the trail meanders through the heart of Irvine.

Kevin Belle

County
Orange

Endpoints
Jamboree Road and Eastbluff Dr. (Newport Beach); Laguna Freeway/ CA 133, south of Alton Pkwy. (Irvine); Dana and Antivo, just south of Dana Park (Irvine)

Mileage
10.8

Type
Greenway/Non-Rail-Trail

Roughness Rating
1

Surface
Asphalt, Concrete

San Diego Creek Trail

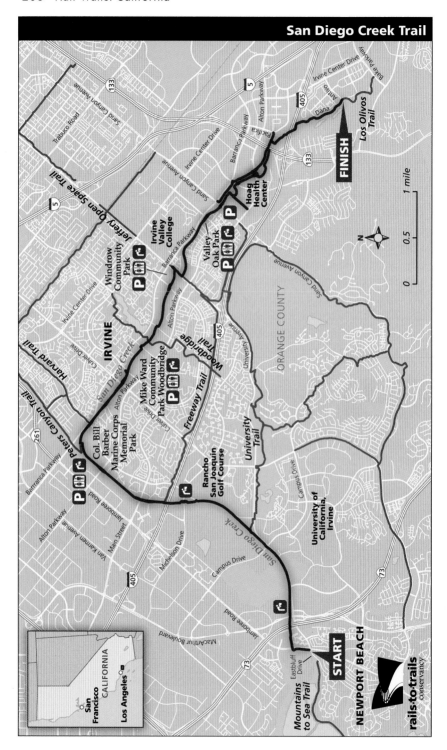

Freeway Trail, Peters Canyon Trail, Harvard Trail, Woodbridge Trail, and Jeffrey Open Space Trail.

Begin your journey at the trail's western endpoint: the northwestern corner of Eastbluff Drive and Jamboree Road in Newport Beach. On-street parking is available on Eastbluff Drive, and a wide sidewalk that's part of the Mountains to Sea Trail serves as a connection to the San Diego Creek Trail. A short section of trail runs alongside Upper Newport Bay, then curves east to begin following San Diego Creek. Continuing northeast along the creek, you pass the Rancho San Joaquin Golf Course before continuing under Michelson Drive and I-405. You'll soon reach Colonel Bill Barber Marine Corps Memorial Park at a bend in the creek, where you'll cross to its north side.

In 2.7 miles, at Windrow Community Park, continue following the trail under Jeffrey Road and turn to cross the creek again to follow the south side (from this point, there are two segments of the trail on either side of the creek). Look out for possible gate closures at roadway intersections; these prevent users from entering segments that may be inaccessible or unsafe due to rising creek waters during heavy rainfall. At Alton Parkway, a short section of trail follows the creek's south side but dead-ends below the Laguna Freeway/CA 133. To end your trip before the San Diego Freeway/I-405, exit the trail via bike lanes on Alton Parkway.

To take the trail to its easternmost endpoint, south of I-405, cross to the north side of the creek at Alton Parkway. Continue on the trail under the Laguna Freeway/CA 133, then continue south under I-405 once again. The trail goes on as the creek turns from a channelized concrete waterway back to a natural creekbed along a subdivision, then ends near Dana and Antivo in Irvine. The trail connects to Los Olivos Trail—a 0.4-mile trail heading south toward Los Olivos Community Park.

CONTACT cityofirvine.org/transportation/irvine-shares-way

continued on next page

PARKING

Parking areas are located within Irvine and are listed from west to east. *Indicates that at least one accessible parking space is available.*

COLONEL BILL BARBER MARINE CORPS MEMORIAL PARK* Harvard Ave. and San Juan (33.6876, -117.8201).

MIKE WARD COMMUNITY PARK WOODBRIDGE* Lake Road, 0.1 mile northeast of Alton Pkwy. (33.6769, -117.8034).

WINDROW COMMUNITY PARK* E. Yale Loop, 400 feet south of Osborn (33.6724, -117.7878).

VALLEY OAK PARK* Valley Oak Dr., between Barranca Pkwy. and Alevera (33.6663, -117.7752).

HOAG HEALTH CENTER 16105 Sand Canyon Ave. (33.6638, -117.7724); enter via the health center complex and take a right toward the end of the parking lot (near power lines) to reach the trail entrance.

Southern California's San Gabriel River Trail extends from the Pacific Ocean to the base of the San Gabriel Mountains, connecting more than a dozen communities east of Los Angeles. The 38-mile paved pathway travels through an exceptionally diverse landscape. In the south, the trail follows the channelized river past a mix of industrial and residential areas, while the northern portion opens up to striking scenic vistas of the surrounding mountains.

Beginning your journey at the trail's southern end, you'll have plentiful amenities at Seal Beach's River's End Park. Heading north, you'll enjoy views of the San Gabriel River to your left. In 2.7 miles, you'll have access to Edison Park, a small, family-friendly spot with a playground and picnic tables, and 2.5 miles beyond that, you'll enter the much larger El Dorado East Regional Park, which offers an archery range, a nature center, fishing lakes, and a plethora of other amenities. Two more parks follow in quick succession: Rynerson Park and Liberty Park, both offering opportunities for various sports.

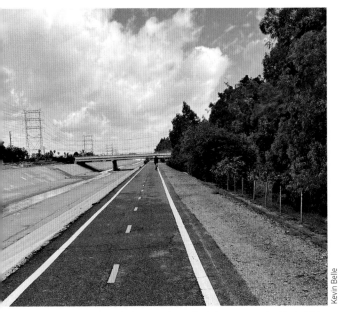

In the south, the trail follows the channelized river past a mix of industrial and residential surroundings.

Kevin Belle

Counties
Los Angeles, Orange

Endpoints
Dead end of First St. at River's End Park (Seal Beach); San Gabriel Canyon Road/CA 39, 1 mile east of Ranch Road (Azusa)

Mileage
38

Type
Greenway/Non-Rail-Trail, Rail-with-Trail

Roughness Rating
1

Surface
Asphalt, Concrete

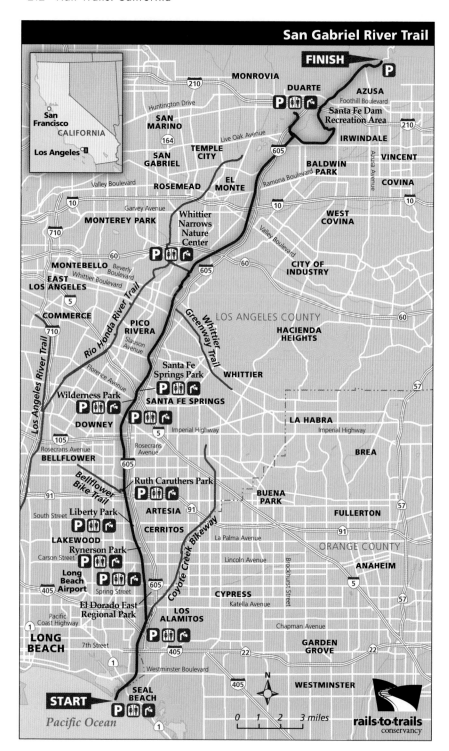

Approaching the trail's midpoint, Santa Fe Springs Park will be your last major stopping point for amenities before a long stretch of open trail with fewer facilities; your next chance for restrooms and drinking water will be at the Whittier Narrows Nature Center, 8 miles farther north. On the trail's northern end, the river returns to its natural course and the pathway passes through scenic protected areas, including the Santa Fe Dam Recreation Area. Be prepared for a short incline at the dam and sun exposure as you explore this drier terrain.

In addition to connecting several parks and natural areas, the trail is also a key component of Los Angeles County's transportation infrastructure. With connections to the Coyote Creek Bikeway, Bellflower Bike Trail, and Rio Hondo River Trail (see page 187), it forms the backbone of a vast trail system for the region. An eventual connection to the Whittier Greenway Trail will provide additional recreational and transportation options.

CONTACT trails.lacounty.gov/trail/265/san-gabriel-river-trail

PARKING

Parking areas are listed from south to north. Select parking areas for the trail are listed below. For a detailed list of parking areas and other waypoints, go to **TrailLink.com**™. *Indicates that at least one accessible parking space is available.*

SEAL BEACH Edison Park, 99 College Park Dr. (33.7754, -118.0966).

LONG BEACH* El Dorado East Regional Park, 7550 E. Spring St. (33.8112, -118.0879).

LAKEWOOD* Rynerson Park, 20711 Studebaker Road (33.8422, -118.0962).

CERRITOS* Liberty Park, 19211 Studebaker Road (33.8537, -118.1011).

BELLFLOWER* Ruth R. Caruthers Park, 10500 E. Flora Vista St. (33.8800, -118.1093).

DOWNEY* Wilderness Park, 10999 Little Lake Road (33.9353, -118.1011).

SANTA FE SPRINGS* Santa Fe Springs Park, 10068 Cedardale Dr. (33.9462, -118.0962).

SOUTH EL MONTE* Whittier Narrows Nature Center, 1000 Durfee Ave. (34.0344, -118.0446).

IRWINDALE* Santa Fe Dam Nature Center, 15501 E. Arrow Hwy. (34.1110, -117.9500).

AZUSA* Azusa Bike Trailhead, 8500–8524 San Gabriel Canyon Road (34.1590, -117.9109).

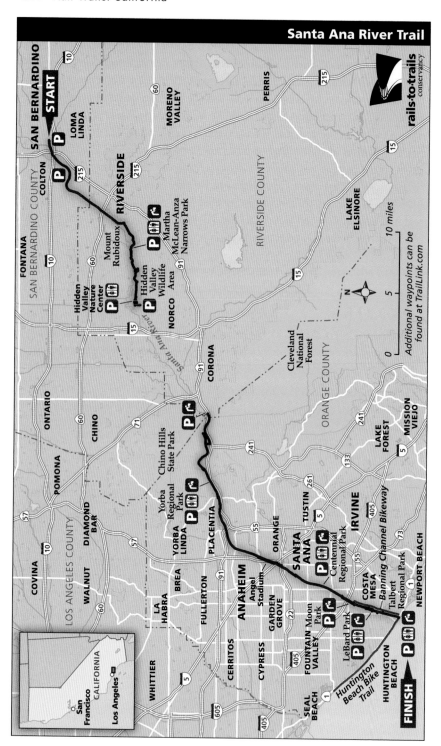

Santa Ana River Trail

rails-to-trails
conservancy

Additional waypoints can be
found at TrailLink.com

The Santa Ana River Trail is a colossus in the emerging greater Los Angeles–area trail network. The paved trail covers nearly 60 miles in two sections, including more than 20 miles through San Bernardino and Riverside Counties and another 30 miles running downstream from Corona all the way through Orange County to the Pacific Ocean. A 7-mile segment in the southern section has trails on both sides of the channel for easier access.

Plans call for extending the trail upriver from San Bernardino through Redlands to the foot of the San Bernardino National Forest, as well as closing the gap between the two existing sections, to complete more than 100 miles of trail. The trail is exposed and can get hot, so dress appropriately, and keep your water bottle full.

The northern section hugs the natural channel as it flows out of the mountains. While there's often little more than a trickle in the riverbed because of diversions for

Counties
San Bernardino, Riverside, Orange

Endpoints
S. Waterman Ave. and E. Hospitality Lane (San Bernardino); Hidden Valley Nature Center at Arlington Ave., 0.5 mile east of Substation Road (Riverside); Green River Road (near CA 91/ Riverside Fwy.), 0.7 mile south of Crestridge Dr. (Corona); Huntington Beach Bike Trail at CA 1/E. Pacific Coast Hwy., 0.4 mile southeast of Brookhurst St. (Huntington Beach)

Mileage
57.7

Type
Greenway/Non-Rail-Trail

Roughness Rating
1

Surface
Asphalt, Concrete

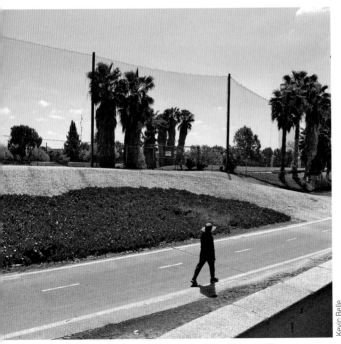

Kevin Belle

The trail offers access to several parks with plentiful amenities and recreational opportunities.

groundwater recharge, flash floods can occur in heavy rains through this arid section. The trail passes under most highway crossings, such as the freeway interchange in San Bernardino, for miles of blissfully uninterrupted travel.

From San Bernardino, the atmosphere becomes quiet and rural, with desert-like vegetation. In about 10 miles, you'll pass the base of Riverside's Mount Rubidoux, a park and prominent feature along the trail. The surroundings become more populated over the next 7 or 8 miles until a short but exhilarating downhill section takes you to the Hidden Valley Wildlife Area, a 1,500-acre, high-desert wildlife sanctuary. There's a nature center here, as well as overlooks of the wide river channel. Birders and horseback riders frequent the area, as do coyotes.

After a 10- to-12-mile gap, the trail begins again in Corona in far-western Riverside County, where a segment across Prado Dam is slated to open in 2025. Beginning again on Green River Road, the trail enters Orange County, where it runs down a mostly concrete channel to the ocean. Transitioning to an urban trail, it passes through the cities of Anaheim, Orange, Santa Ana, and others.

Along the way, ramps to road crossings allow trail users to exit the channel and explore area dining, shopping, or parkland. In northern Orange County, Yorba Regional Park has 400 picnic tables scattered among the trees and lakesides. The Los Angeles Angels play at the Anaheim stadium complex about 9 miles downriver, and Talbert Regional Park in Costa Mesa features different groupings of vegetation found along the river.

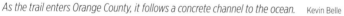

As the trail enters Orange County, it follows a concrete channel to the ocean.   Kevin Belle

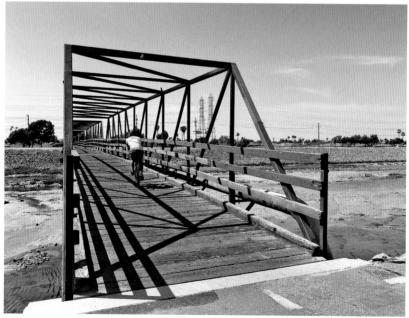

The trail connects seamlessly to the Huntington Beach Bicycle Trail (see page 95), which rolls up the coast for 8 miles of beaches in Surf City USA. It also connects to the Banning Channel Bikeway, which travels up the east side of the Santa Ana channel for 3 miles to Costa Mesa.

CONTACT rtc.li/santa-ana-sbcounty and rivcoparks.org/santa-ana-river-trail

PARKING

Parking areas are listed from north to south. Select parking areas for the trail are listed below. For a detailed list of parking areas and other waypoints, go to **TrailLink.com**™. *Indicates that at least one accessible parking space is available.*

NORTHERN SEGMENT

SAN BERNARDINO* County office parking, S. Hunts Lane, 0.2 mile north W. Hospitality Lane (34.0685, -117.2885)

COLTON S. La Cadena Dr. at W. Tropica Rancho Road (34.0441, -117.3320).

RIVERSIDE* Martha McLean–Anza Narrows Park, 5759 Jurupa Ave. (33.9658, -117.4321).

RIVERSIDE* Hidden Valley Nature Center, Hidden Valley Nature Center Road, 1.5 miles north of Arlington Ave. (33.9611, -117.4959).

RIVERSIDE Hidden Valley Wilderness Area, Arlington Ave. and Hidden Valley Nature Center Road (33.9551, -117.5143).

SOUTHERN SEGMENT

CORONA* Trailhead, 4995 Green River Road, 0.8 mile west of Exit 44 off CA 91/ Riverside Fwy. (33.8712, -117.6684).

ANAHEIM* Yorba Regional Park, La Palma Ave., 0.1 mile northwest of Fairmont Blvd. (33.8656, -117.7732).

SANTA ANA* Centennial Regional Park, Edinger Dr. and S. Mohawk Dr. (33.7267, -117.9127).

COSTA MESA* Moon Park, 3377 California St., at Nevada Ave. (33.6941, -117.9336).

HUNTINGTON BEACH* LeBard Park, Warwick Dr., between Ravenswood Lane and Craimer Lane (33.6653, -117.9498).

HUNTINGTON BEACH* Huntington State Beach, CA 1/E. Pacific Coast Hwy. at Brookhurst St. (33.6339, -117.9626).

Santa Fe Trail

The 19th-century railroad-building boom brought the town of Tulare into existence in California's Central Valley. More than 100 years later, the town transformed a former railroad spur into the Santa Fe Trail, which connects residential areas on both ends with the downtown commercial district.

The 5-mile paved trail takes an east–west route that is as flat as the surrounding valley; the only exception is the ramp up to a pedestrian bridge that crosses an active railroad line. Much of the trail, except through downtown, is accompanied by a bridle path separated by a fence.

The valley is cloudy and cool in the winter but hot as blazes in the summer. You will find about a dozen drinking fountains to quench your thirst along the way, or you can escape the heat by strolling beneath the streetlights that illuminate the trail at night through downtown. Although there's no leafy canopy, trees planted along the corridor offer occasional shade.

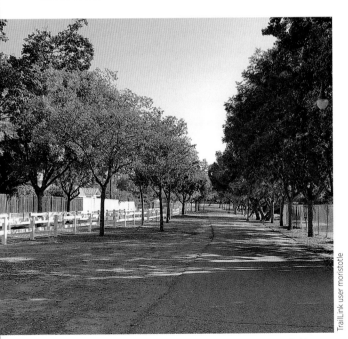

Much of the trail, except through downtown Tulare, is accompanied by a fenced-off bridle path.

TrailLink user moristotle

County
Tulare

Endpoints
E. Prosperity Ave.,
0.4 mile east of
N. Mooney Blvd. (Tulare);
W. Inyo Ave./CA 137
and W. Soults Dr.

Mileage
5

Type
Rail-Trail

Roughness Rating
1

Surface
Asphalt, Dirt

The town was founded in 1872 as a regional headquarters for the Southern Pacific Railroad. It was named for nearby Tulare Lake, whose name comes from the tules (bulrushes) that the Indigenous people of the area fashioned into reed boats and more for centuries. The lake has since dried up, and the town faced a similar fate when the railroad headquarters moved away. Instead, the town built canals and adopted other dry-land agricultural practices that have made the area a dairy industry leader.

The trail follows a spur line once operated by the Atchison, Topeka and Santa Fe Railway. It opened in 2004, 10 years after the railroad ceased operations. Popular for recreation, the trail also runs within a half mile of virtually all of Tulare's schools to enable safe student travel.

Starting at the northeast edge of town on Prosperity Avenue, you'll notice a separate, fenced horse path paralleling the paved trail. This dirt path goes 2.2 miles to North Cherry Street, then resumes on the other side of downtown for a 0.9-mile run between North West Street and the trail's terminus at West Inyo Avenue/CA 137.

One mile from the starting point, the trail arrives at Live Oak Park, where you'll find parking, ball fields, restrooms, and picnic shelters. In another half mile, you'll cross over the busy Golden State Highway/CA 99, then go another mile to downtown, with its variety of restaurants, bus station, and library, among other amenities.

To take the pedestrian overpass across an active rail line, cross North K Street, go a half block north, and then turn left at the sidewalk that leads to the ramp. You'll pick up the trail on North I Street and continue west through a residential area about 2 miles until the trail ends at West Inyo Avenue/CA 137.

CONTACT rtc.li/city-tulare

PARKING

Parking areas are located within Tulare and are listed from east to west. *Indicates that at least one accessible parking space is available.*

LIVE OAK PARK* 600 N. Laspina St. (36.2174, -119.3206).
MUNICIPAL PARKING* 463 N. J St., between E. Cross Ave. and E. San Joaquin Ave. (36.2124, -119.3481).

The Stevens Creek Trail runs through the heart of Silicon Valley on two disconnected sections in Mountain View and Cupertino. The trail offers access to, and views of, the tech world's premier campuses while providing a welcome off-street, multiuse corridor for the densely populated communities. Parks on both ends of the trail (Stevens Creek Shoreline Nature Study Area Preserve in the north and McClellan Ranch Preserve and Blackberry Farm in the south) are popular destinations for recreation and learning about local wildlife along the creek.

The trail and the creek are named after Captain Elijah Stevens, a blacksmith and leader of the first wagon train of settlers to cross the Sierra Nevada during the westward expansion of the 1840s. Regarded as one of the better-preserved creeks in the Bay Area, the creek has retained much of its natural channel, flowing from the Santa Cruz Mountains and through Stevens Canyon before eventually

County
Santa Clara

Endpoints
Bay Trail at Stevens Creek Shoreline Nature Study Area Preserve, 1.8 mile north of US 101/Bayshore Fwy.; Dale Ave. and Heatherstone Way (Mountain View); Blackberry Farm Golf Course, Stevens Creek Blvd., between Cupertino Road and Phar Lap Dr. (Cupertino); Linda Vista Park at Linda Vista Dr., 300 feet south of Columbus Ave. (Cupertino)

Mileage
5.9

Type
Greenway/Non-Rail-Trail

Roughness Rating
1

Surface
Asphalt

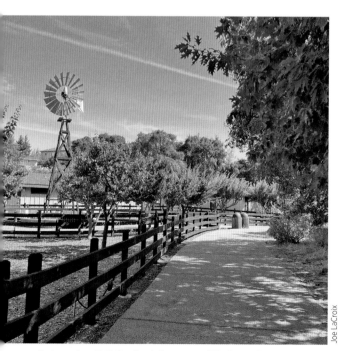

Joe LaCroix

Parks, such as McClellan Ranch Preserve and Blackberry Farm, are popular destinations along the trail.

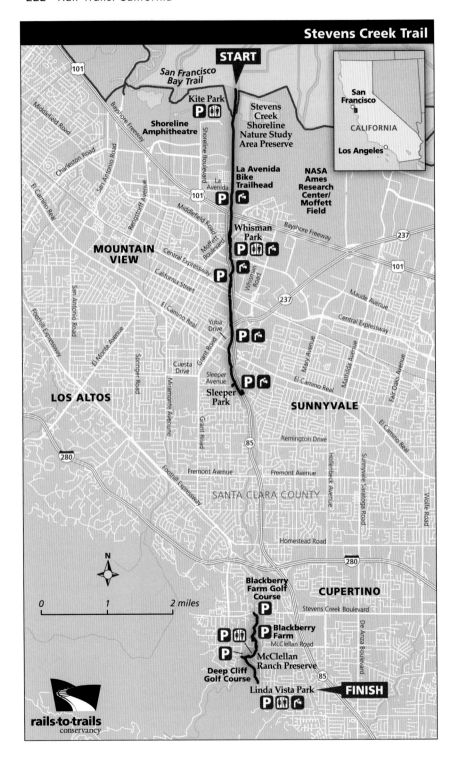

Stevens Creek Trail

START

101

San Francisco
Bay Trail

Kite Park
P 🚻

Shoreline
Amphitheatre

Stevens
Creek
Shoreline
Nature Study
Area Preserve

San
Francisco

CALIFORNIA

Los Angeles

Shoreline Boulevard

La Avenida
Bike
Trailhead
P 🚲

La
Avenida

101

Middlefield Road

NASA
Ames
Research
Center/
Moffett
Field

Middlefield Road

Charleston Road

Bayshore Freeway

San Antonio Road

Rengstorff Avenue

Moffett Boulevard

Whisman
Park
P 🚻 🚲

237

101

MOUNTAIN
VIEW

Central Expressway

California Street

El Camino Real

Whisman Road

237

Maude Avenue

El Camino Real

San Antonio Road

P

Yuba
Drive

P 🚲

Central Expressway

El Monte Avenue

Springer Road

Cuesta
Drive

Grant Road

Sleeper
Avenue

P 🚲

Mary Avenue

Mathilda Avenue

Fair Oaks Avenue

El Camino Real

LOS ALTOS

Miramonte Avenue

Sleeper
Park

SUNNYVALE

El Camino Real

280

Grant Road

85

Remington Drive

Hollenbeck Avenue

Sunnyvale Saratoga Road

Wolfe Road

Foothill Expressway

Fremont Avenue

Fremont Avenue

SANTA CLARA COUNTY

Homestead Road

N

280

0   1   2 miles

Blackberry
Farm Golf
Course
P

CUPERTINO

Stevens Creek Boulevard

De Anza Boulevard

P 🚻

P Blackberry
Farm

McClellan Road

P

McClellan
Ranch Preserve

85

Deep Cliff
Golf Course

Linda Vista Park
P 🚻 🚲

FINISH

rails·to·trails
conservancy

emptying into the southern end of the San Francisco Bay. Sections of trail pass through forested foothills, lowland creeks, and marshy protected wetlands.

The northern segment in Mountain View, about 5 miles long, begins near a junction with the San Francisco Bay Trail, a developing network of 500 miles of trails encircling the bay. Both the Stevens Creek Trail and the San Francisco Bay Trail are part of a developing 2,600-miles-plus Bay Area regional trail network being spearheaded by the Bay Area Trails Collaborative (**railstotrails.org/bay -area**) and Rails-to-Trails Conservancy as a TrailNation™ project to increase safe walking, biking, and trail access for millions of Bay Area residents.

Coursing southward from the 750-acre nature preserve, the trail runs through tidal marshlands juxtaposed against the uniquely modern architecture of the tech-giant campuses. After you leave the park, grade-separated crossings of busy roads allow for uninterrupted travel to the trail's endpoint in a residential sector of Mountain View at Heatherstone Way and Dale Avenue. Multiple bike repair stations can be found along this section. The cities of Mountain View and Sunnyvale have planned to extend the trail about 2 miles from here.

In Cupertino, a 1.3-mile stretch of the Stevens Creek Trail links two popular community parks. The first, Blackberry Farm, offers ample picnic space, swimming pools, a playground, and many other amenities and runs alongside

The trail runs through Silicon Valley, with views of the tech world's premier campuses, such as Google's Bay View campus, shown here.   Joe LaCroix

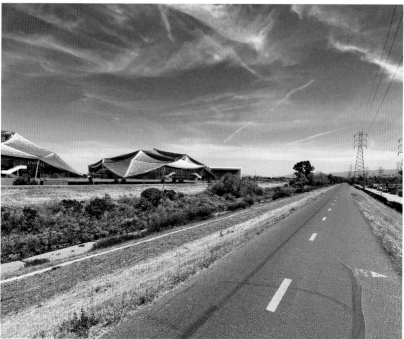

a public golf course. The McClellan Ranch Preserve, a charming horse ranch contains a nature museum; a community garden; and a petting zoo with friendly alpacas, goats, and other farm animals. The ranch offers ample parking, as well as restrooms and water.

Across McClellan Road, the trail passes alongside the Deep Cliff Golf Course, ending at Linda Vista Park, where you'll find restrooms, picnic areas, playgrounds, and other recreational activities. The Linda Vista Park section of trail, loosely paved and with steep elevation changes, is not recommended for wheelchair users.

CONTACT stevenscreektrail.org

PARKING

Parking areas are listed from north to south. *Indicates that at least one accessible parking space is available.*

MOUNTAIN VIEW SEGMENT

KITE PARK* N. Shoreline Blvd, 0.1 mile north of North Road, 0.7 mile east of Stevens Creek Trail (37.4299, -122.0772).

LA AVENIDA BIKE TRAILHEAD La Avenida St., 0.2 mile east of Armand Dr. (37.4129, -122.0691).

WHISMAN PARK* Easy St., 0.1 mile north of E. Middlefield Road (37.4003, -122.0661).

CENTRAL AVE. TRAILHEAD 101–195 Central Ave., 240 feet southeast of Orchard Ave. (37.3950, -122.0697).

YUBA DR. TRAILHEAD 715 Yuba Dr., at Church St. (37.3824, -122.0686).

SLEEPER AVE. TRAILHEAD Sleeper Ave. and Franklin Ave. (37.3716, -122.0683); on-street parking.

CUPERTINO SEGMENT

BLACKBERRY FARM GOLF COURSE* 22100 Stevens Creek Blvd. (37.3227, -122.0599); the trailhead is about 0.1 mile west of the parking lot.

BLACKBERRY FARM* 21979 San Fernando Ave. (37.3183, -122.0608).

MCCLELLAN RANCH PRESERVE* McClellan Road, 0.1 mile east of Club House Lane (37.3131, -122.0635).

LINDA VISTA PARK* Linda Vista Dr., 0.1 mile south of Columbus Ave. (37.3074, -122.0603)

For more than 50 years in the early 1900s, the Sugar Pine Railway operated steam trains to haul logs along the Stanislaus River for the Standard Lumber Company and, later, the Pickering Lumber Company. Today, this wooded corridor, sometimes called the Strawberry Branch, hosts a gentle, 3% grade rail-trail for hikers, mountain bikers, and cross-country skiers (while open to equestrians, the trail is rarely used by them due to limited parking and access for horse trailers). The trail represents a very small part of the Sugar Pine Railway system, which included about 70 miles of main line and almost 400 miles of spurs and branches. While there are a number of rail-trails in the Sierra left over from the area's extensive logging history, this is one of the easiest and most family-friendly because of its accessibility, gentle grade, and relatively forgiving dirt surface.

Interpretive signs along the trail point out historical highlights and trailside features. The signs are numbered

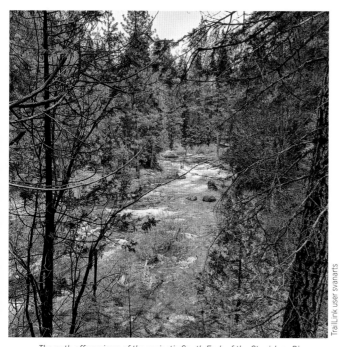

The path offers views of the majestic South Fork of the Stanislaus River.

TrailLink user svanarts

County
Tuolumne

Endpoints
Fraser Flat Road at South Fork of Stanislaus River (Long Barn); Old Strawberry Road (Pinecrest)

Mileage
2.5

Type
Rail-Trail

Roughness Rating
2–3

Surface
Dirt

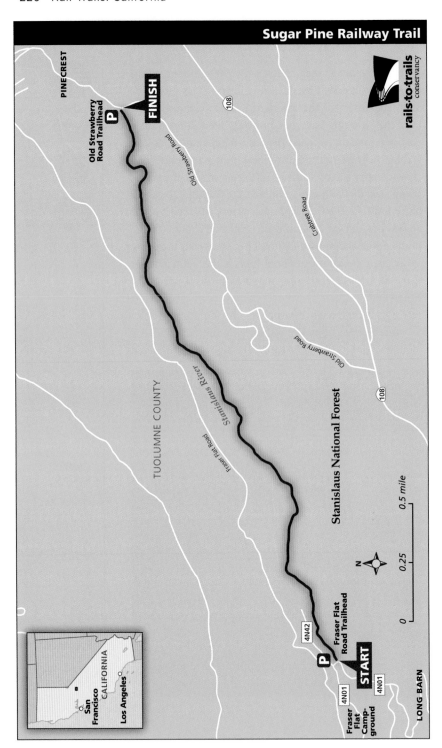

Sugar Pine Railway Trail

for use with an informational brochure that you can pick up from the Summit Ranger Station (1 Pinecrest Lake Road) in Pinecrest—only a 6.7-mile drive from the Fraser Flat Road Trailhead—or the Stanislaus National Forest Supervisor's Office (19777 Greenley Road) in Sonora—more than 25 miles south of the Fraser Flat Road Trailhead. It's a good idea to also pick up a map of the area, as the roads are not well marked and finding your way around can be challenging. Along those lines, it can be difficult to find the Old Strawberry Road Trailhead, as signage is minimal.

Start at the Fraser Flat Road Trailhead in Long Barn for a nicely shaded, gradual uphill grade that affords great views of the majestic South Fork of the Stanislaus River below. (*Note:* There are no restrooms or potable water along the trail, so be sure to plan accordingly.) The dirt trail surface can be loose in places, and there are some considerable dips in the trail, so be careful and keep your eye on what's ahead. At the 1.5-mile mark, you'll pass through an unlocked cattle fence. When the trail opens up into a meadow, look across the meadow to see where the trail reenters the forest.

The trail ends when it intersects Old Strawberry Road. Your return trip on the trail to Long Barn is downhill. In the winter, a cross-country ski route is accessible from the northeastern end of the trail in Pinecrest.

CONTACT fs.usda.gov/recarea/stanislaus/recarea/?recid=15083

PARKING

Parking areas are listed from west to east. *Indicates that at least one accessible parking space is available.*

LONG BARN* Fraser Flat Road Trailhead, FR 4N01 and FR 4N42, adjacent to the South Fork of the Stanislaus River on the south side of the road, 0.5 mile east of Fraser Flat Campground (38.1722, -120.0621).; roadside dirt parking for 4–5 vehicles. Note that FR 4N01, which leads to the Fraser Flat Road Trailhead, is closed starting at CA 108 from mid-December to mid-April.

PINECREST* Old Strawberry Road Trailhead, west side of Old Strawberry Road, 2 miles northeast of CA 108 and Crabtree Road (38.1867, -120.0193); roadside dirt pullouts for 2–3 vehicles. While Old Strawberry Road and the trail from this end are plowed of snow during the winter and reachable year-round, the parking area itself is not plowed.

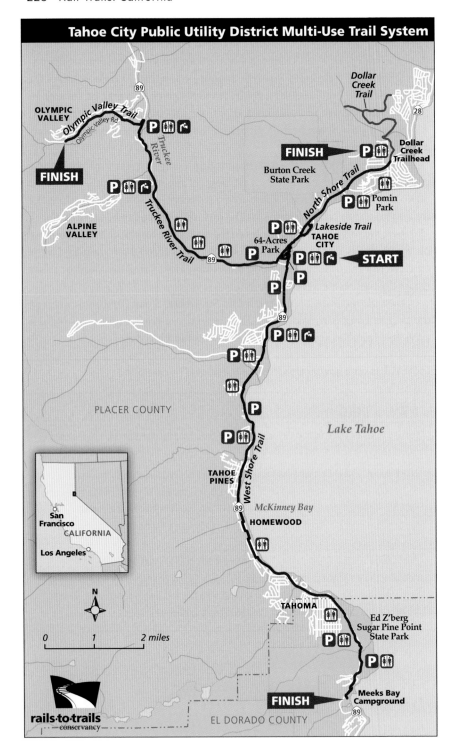

Tahoe City Public Utility District Multi-Use Trail System

The Tahoe City Public Utility District (TCPUD) Multi-Use Trail System meanders along the scenic west shore of Lake Tahoe and weaves through pine and aspen trees along the Truckee River. This 19-mile trail system, previously known as Tahoe Trailways, offers visitors the opportunity to explore Tahoe's lush landscape in three directions: west to Olympic Valley along the Truckee River and Olympic Valley Trails, north to Dollar Creek along the North Shore and Lakeside Trails, or south to Meeks Bay along the West Shore Trail.

The trail consists of two lanes of paved asphalt and offers amenities throughout, including restrooms, water fountains, and picnic areas—many shaded. The trail is plowed in the wintertime. Trailside signs advise walkers and runners to stay on the left side of the trail and cyclists to use the right side, so be cautious while passing in either direction. There is a speed limit of 15 miles per hour for all users throughout the network.

The trail system's vortex is 64-Acres Park, at the intersection of CA 89 and CA 28 in downtown Tahoe City.

Counties
El Dorado, Placer

Endpoints
64-Acres Park, CA 89/
W. Lake Blvd. and CA 28/
W. River Road (Tahoe
City); Christy Hill Road
and Olympic Valley
Road (Olympic Valley);
CA 89/N. Lake Blvd. and
Dollar Dr. (Tahoe City);
Meeks Campground
at Emerald Bay Road
(Tahoma)

Mileage
18.7

Type
Rail-Trail, Greenway

Roughness Rating
1

Surface
Asphalt

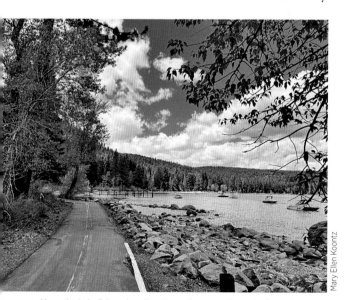

Mary Ellen Koontz

Along the Lake Tahoe shoreline, the path weaves through pine and aspen trees.

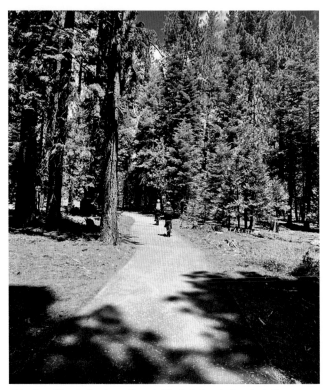

Tahoe's multiuse trail system offers a brilliantly lush and often shaded landscape.
Mary Ellen Koontz

Heading north along the Lakeside Trail, you'll pass shops, dining, and lodging. The trail passes through the Commons Beach lakefront picnic area, which has restrooms, bike racks, a playground, and a bike repair station, before continuing north along the North Shore Trail. The trail runs parallel to CA 28 and passes through residential areas en route to the northern terminus at Dollar Creek, where visitors can connect to the 2.2-mile Dollar Creek Trail.

Venturing west from 64-Acres Park, you'll follow the Truckee River Trail 5.5 miles to Olympic Park in Olympic Valley, site of the 1960 Winter Olympics. This path weaves among towering conifers along the corridor of the former Lake Tahoe Railway and Transportation Company, which operated from the early 1900s until 1943. In the summer, the Truckee River is a popular kayaking, fishing, and rafting destination. At Olympic Valley Road, the trail connects to the Olympic Valley Trail, which heads 2.1 miles west to the ski resort.

If you choose to head south along the West Shore Trail, you'll be treated to tree-lined trails and dazzling views of Lake Tahoe along the system's longest branch at nearly 11 miles. The trail mostly hugs the lake, running parallel to CA 89, with some on-road routes through adjacent neighborhoods between 64-Acres Park and Ed Z'berg Sugar Pine Point State Park. Crossings are well marked with signs and signals to vehicular traffic. As you descend to the southern terminus at Meeks Bay Campground, take time to enjoy the breathtaking views of the lake and surrounding Sierra Nevada.

CONTACT tcpud.org/trails

PARKING

Parking areas are listed by trail. Select parking areas for the trail are listed below. For a detailed list of parking areas and other waypoints, go to **TrailLink.com**™. *Indicates that at least one accessible parking space is available.*

LAKESIDE AND NORTH SHORE TRAILS (south to north)

TAHOE CITY* 64-Acres Park, W. Lake Blvd. and CA 89/Lake Blvd. (39.1642, -120.1474).

TAHOE CITY Commons Beach, Commons Beach Road at CA 28/N. Lake Blvd. (39.1693, -120.1421).

TAHOE CITY* Pomin Park, 2500 Lake Forest Road (39.1826, -120.1201).

TAHOE CITY* Dollar Creek Trailhead, CA 28/N. Lake Blvd. and Dollar Dr. (39.1938, -120.1046). Heading north on CA 28/N. Lake Blvd., you'll turn left into the entrance to the parking lot. The North Shore Trail's northern endpoint is at the turn, where CA 28/N. Lake Blvd. meets Dollar Dr.

TRUCKEE RIVER TRAIL (east to west)

TAHOE CITY* Bells Landing, CA 89/River Road, 0.3 mile south of Alpine Meadows Road (39.1839, -120.1955).

OLYMPIC VALLEY Olympic Valley Park, Olympic Valley Road, 0.1 mile west of CA 89/ River Road (39.2045, -120.2011).

WEST SHORE TRAIL (north to south)

TAHOE CITY* Community Center, Granlibakken Road, just west of CA.89/W. Lake Blvd. (39.1612, -120.1468).

TAHOE CITY* Rideout Community Center, 740 Timberland Lane, 0.2 mile west of CA 89/W. Lake Blvd. (39.1291, -120.1655).

TAHOMA* Ed Z'berg Sugar Pine Point State Park, State Park Road, 0.2 mile east of CA 89/W. Lake Blvd. (39.0501, -120.1147); a fee is charged.

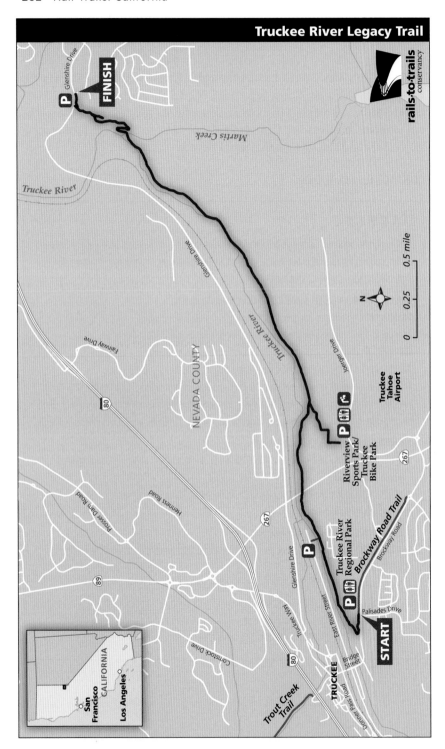

The Truckee River Legacy Trail follows its namesake river's south side from downtown Truckee to the Glenshire neighborhood. The trail provides scenic views of the Truckee River and the High Sierra Crest. Access to several parks, as well as picnic tables, benches, and interpretive signage, is available throughout the route. The trail is popular among hikers, cyclists, birders, and fishers. The State of California, which has designated portions of the Truckee River as Wild Trout Water, manages nearly 11 miles of stream habitat to sustain wild trout species and provide recreational fishing. The Truckee River Legacy Trail is part of the Tahoe–Pyramid Bikeway, which connects trails and on-road routes between Lake Tahoe and Pyramid Lake in Nevada.

The trail's current western endpoint is in Truckee River Regional Park. (The Town of Truckee is extending the trail westward. Once complete, the trail will run from Donner Memorial State Park to its current eastern endpoint on Glenshire Drive.) Start at the south end of the park at the intersection of Palisades Drive and Old

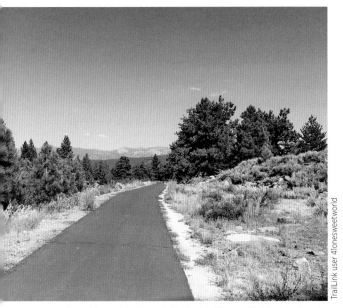

The trail provides scenic views of the Truckee River and High Sierra Crest.

TrailLink user 4lonesweetworld

County
Nevada

Endpoints
S./SE River St. and Palisades Dr. (Truckee); Glenshire Dr. and Berkshire Cir. (Truckee)

Mileage
4.8

Type
Greenway/Non-Rail-Trail

Roughness Rating
1

Surface
Asphalt

Brockway Road. At this signed intersection, take a left to follow a paved trail that heads west, makes a switchback, and then heads north farther into the park. This intersection also marks the start of the Brockway Road Trail, which heads 1 mile southeast and connects to additional trails in Martis Valley.

At 62 acres, Truckee River Regional Park features a ride-on miniature train, a disc golf course, gravel hiking trails, a rentable picnic shelter, river access, restrooms, and the region's oldest man-made structure: the Stampede Circle of Stones. At least 500 years old, the circle was built by the Washoe or their predecessors, the Martis people, in Stampede Valley. The circle was moved to the regional park in 1969, shortly before construction of a dam flooded the valley.

After 1.9 miles, you have the option of taking a brief 0.4-mile spur to Riverview Sports Park. To enter the park, simply take a sharp right at the fork in the trail. Once back on the Truckee River Legacy Trail, you'll travel another 2.9 miles to the trail's eastern endpoint at Glenshire Drive, just before the Glenshire neighborhood sign. This segment includes a bridge over Martis Creek.

For trail users opting for a one-way trip, rather than an out-and-back, start from the westernmost endpoint and head east, as there is a significant uphill grade heading west from Glenshire Drive. Trail users seeking no grade issues are advised to begin their journey at the pedestrian bridge at East River Street and head east. A bike repair station also is available at East River Street.

Also originating in downtown Truckee is the 1.5-mile Trout Creek Trail, a paved trail heading northwest to the Tahoe Donner neighborhood.

CONTACT townoftruckee.com/government/truckee-trails-and-bikeways

---

PARKING

Parking areas are located within Truckee and are listed from west to east. *Indicates that at least one accessible parking space is available.*

TRUCKEE RIVER REGIONAL PARK* 10500 Old Brockway Road (39.3275, -120.1758).

E. RIVER ST.* Parking is adjacent to the pedestrian bridge at the east end of the street; cross the bridge over the Truckee River to reach the trail (39.3313, -120.1689).

TRUCKEE BIKE PARK* 12180 Joerger Dr. (39.3282, -120.1526).

GLENSHIRE DR.* 0.1 mile west of Berkshire Cir. and 0.3 mile south of Old State Route 40 (39.3544, -120.1147); includes two designated van-accessible spaces.

The spectacular Valley Loop Trail is steeped in history and beauty. This easy, paved pathway takes you past some of the most beautiful spots in Yosemite National Park and follows some of Yosemite Valley's historical footpaths and wagon roads. The multiuse trail can become very crowded during peak tourist months in the summer. For a less crowded experience, visit during the shoulder seasons: after the snow has melted or just prior to the snow beginning. The National Park Service practices a simple "pedal to pavement" rule when it comes to biking in Yosemite National Park, meaning that if a trail is not paved, you are not allowed to ride it.

The eastern portion of the Valley Loop Trail, described here, covers 7.5 miles. Start at the Yosemite Valley Visitor

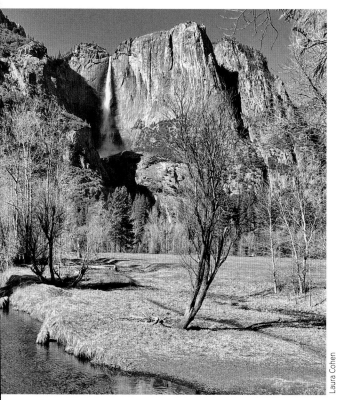

Laura Cohen

The pathway takes you past some of the most beautiful spots in Yosemite National Park.

County
Mariposa

Endpoints
Yosemite Valley Visitor Center (Yosemite Valley); Mirror Lake Trail, 0.4 mile north of Yosemite Shuttle Stop #17 (Yosemite Valley); Happy Isle Loop Road (Yosemite Valley)

Mileage
7.5

Type
Greenway/Non-Rail-Trail

Roughness Rating
1

Surface
Asphalt

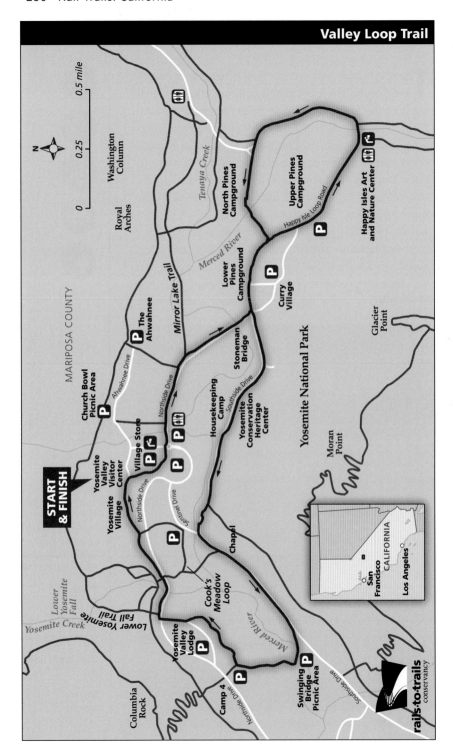

Center, the best place for information about current trail conditions. Pick up a map while you're there, as signage along the trail is somewhat lacking. Just 0.1 mile east of the visitor center, you have the option of taking a scenic 0.6-mile spur following Ahwahnee Drive, ending at the iconic Ahwahnee hotel, built in 1927 and a designated National Historic Landmark.

After you return from the spur, take the trail southeast as it weaves through Yosemite Village, paralleling Northside Drive on the north side of the road. Around 0.4 mile from a roundabout at Village and Northside Drives, you can either continue southeast along Northside Drive or head east toward Mirror Lake Trail, a hiking-only path. Continuing 0.3 mile southeast along Northside Drive, you will come to Stoneman Bridge; be ready with your camera to capture its views of the Merced River.

After the bridge, turn left to head east for a 1.7-mile loop along a shared pedestrian/bicycle lane on Happy Isle Loop Road. Near the northern end of the loop is the southern trailhead of the Mirror Lake Trail. Continuing west to Southside Drive, the trail alternates between the southern and northern sides of the road.

The trail turns north at the Swinging Bridge picnic area, where there is a lovely beach for a cool swim in the Merced River. Cross the river again, following the trail north to Northside Drive. Just 0.8 mile from the picnic area is the start of a trail to Lower Yosemite Fall, part of North America's tallest waterfall, but use caution, as there may be lots of other people along this popular pathway.

After visiting the waterfall, follow the trail east along the north side of Northside Drive. In 0.2 mile, the Valley Loop Trail connects to the Cook's Meadow Loop. Continue east along the Valley Loop Trail another 0.4 mile to return to the visitor center.

CONTACT nps.gov/yose/planyourvisit/valleylooptrail.htm

continued on next page

PARKING

Parking areas are located within Yosemite Valley and are listed clockwise. Note that parking areas throughout the national park are very congested in the summer, and entrance fees apply. For information on transportation in and around the park, visit **nps.gov/yose/planyourvisit /publictransportation.htm.** Select parking areas for the trail are listed below. For a detailed list of parking areas and other waypoints, go to **TrailLink.com™.** *Indicates that at least one accessible parking space is available.*

VILLAGE STORE* 9011 Village Dr. (37.7470, -119.5846).

CHURCH BOWL PICNIC AREA* 9000 Ahwahnee Dr. (37.7486, -119.5810).

THE AHWAHNEE* 1 Ahwahnee Dr. (37.7472, -119.5746).

CURRY VILLAGE CAMPGROUND RESERVATION OFFICE* 9024 Southside Dr. (37.7385, -119.5697).

YOSEMITE VALLEY TRAILHEAD Dead end of Happy Isle Loop Road, 0.6 mile southeast of Southside Dr. (37.7351, -119.5671); gravel lot.

SWINGING BRIDGE PICNIC AREA* Southside Dr., 2 miles northeast of El Capitan Dr. (37.7366, -119.5994).

NORTHSIDE DR.* Northside Dr., 0.9 mile southwest of Village Dr. (37.7411, -119.6016).

YOSEMITE VALLEY LODGE* 9006 Yosemite Lodge Dr. (37.7436, -119.5982).

SENTINEL DR.* Sentinel Dr., 0.1 mile north of Southside Dr., Yosemite Shuttle Stop #11 (37.7440, -119.5898).

YOSEMITE VILLAGE PARKING* Northside Dr., between Sentinel Dr. and the roundabout at Village Dr. and Northside Dr. (37.7441, -119.5850).

The Ventura River Trail follows the former Southern Pacific Railroad right-of-way from the entrance of Foster Park south to the city of Ventura. The trail has a distinctly industrial feel, giving trail users a close-up look at the many businesses (past and present) that have fueled the region's growth. Opened in 1999, the Ventura River Trail continues north to the city of Ojai as the Ojai Valley Trail.

Start your journey at Foster Park, a lovely linear county park and a popular barbecue spot on weekends and holidays. You'll be paralleling CA 33/Ojai Freeway and North Ventura Avenue, but the roads are not always visible from the trail. Heading south from the northern endpoint, you'll reach a trailhead in about 0.4 mile, just before North Ventura Avenue crosses beneath CA 33/Ojai Freeway. This portion of the trail winds along pastureland and an equestrian path, with the Ventura River on one side and North Ventura Avenue on the other.

By the time you reach the trail's midpoint, the scenery transitions as you pass a variety of features from the area's

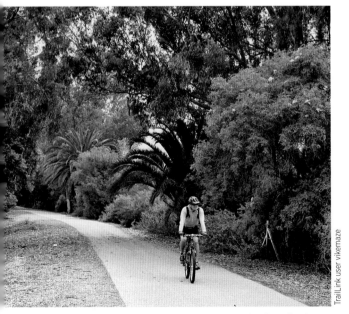

TrailLink user vikemaze

Although largely an urban experience, there are occasional tree-lined sections of trail.

County
Ventura

Endpoints
Ojai Valley Trail at Casitas Vista Road (Ventura); Rex St. and Dubbers St. (Ventura)

Mileage
5.5

Type
Rail-Trail

Roughness Rating
1

Surface
Asphalt

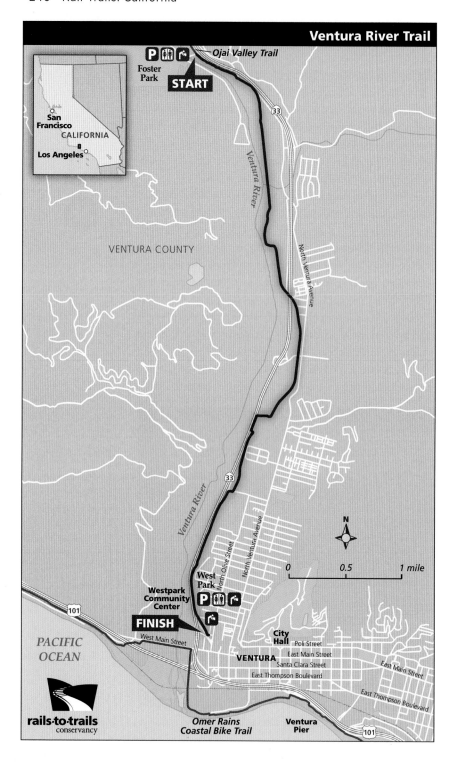

natural and industrial heritage, including an impressive wall of sedimentary layers exposed by the Ventura River, active and abandoned industrial sites, and the occasional oil derrick. It may not be the most scenic stretch of trail, but it is certainly interesting. The route is also marked by a series of art installations incorporating themes related to Ventura, including *Orange Trace,* which features clusters of painted bronze oranges arranged to look like they just fell from a freight car.

Your journey ends in Ventura (officially San Buenaventura). If you're visiting the city for the first time, you might want to check out any number of sites. Ventura's City Hall, a 1912 marble and terra-cotta Beaux Arts building, evokes memories of a long-gone era of the Central Coast. The Ventura Pier, built in 1872, is Southern California's second-oldest pier and a great place to watch surfers catching waves.

The trail is paved and in good condition, crossing roads occasionally. Bicycle and pedestrian traffic is fairly light in spring but picks up in summer. Like most rail-trails, the Ventura River Trail is a very comfortable ride, though there is a slight uphill grade if you double back and head north to Foster Park.

Trail users seeking to enjoy a spectacular downhill bike ride can start in downtown Ojai and follow the Ojai Valley Trail (see page 165) and Ventura River Trail. Arriving in Ventura, turn right on North Olive Street and right on North Main Street to meet the Omer Rains Coastal Bike Trail just past CA 33/ Ojai Freeway. Turn left to follow it to the Ventura Pier and the Pacific Coast.

CONTACT www.cityofventura.ca.gov/420/Bicycling-Walking

PARKING

Parking areas are located within Ventura and are listed from north to south. *Indicates that at least one accessible parking space is available.*

FOSTER PARK* Day-Use Area, paved lot at roundabout at the northern end of Ventura River Area, 0.3 mile north of 59 Casitas Vista Road (34.3567, -119.3097).

WESTPARK COMMUNITY CENTER* 450 W. Harrison Ave. (34.2874, -119.3055).

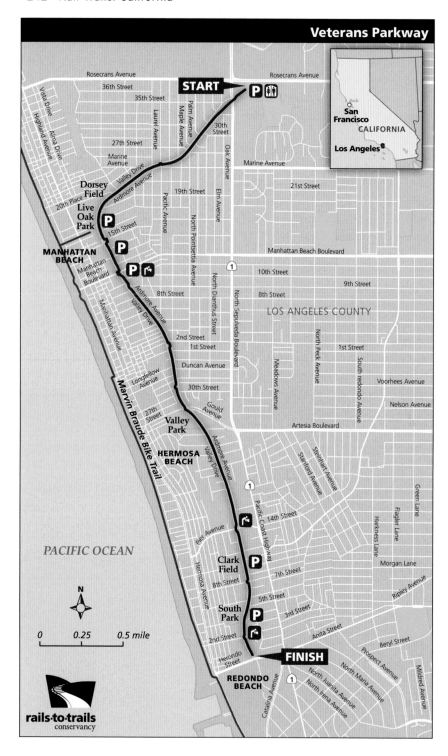

Joggers and walkers using the 3.5-mile Veterans Parkway trail through the beach towns of Hermosa Beach and Manhattan Beach should never go hungry.

The soft-surface pedestrian-only trail (no bikes or horses) passes numerous shops selling coffee and lemonade, as well as pancakes, pizza, and burritos, as it runs the length of the two towns sandwiched between Redondo Beach in the south and El Segundo in the north. Much of it runs within a half mile of popular Pacific beaches.

Formerly known as the Hermosa Valley Greenbelt, the corridor got its start in 1888 as a branch line of the Santa Fe Railway to haul goods to and from the wharves at Redondo Beach. Freight shipping declined after a major port opened elsewhere in 1909, and passenger service ended in 1918 due to competition from electric trolleys. The two beach towns separately acquired their segments of the disused rail corridor in the late 1980s and, after referenda and lawsuits, settled on creating a trail along the towns' only greenbelt a few years later.

County
Los Angeles

Endpoints
Access road 450 feet south of Rosecrans Ave., near CA 1/N. Sepulveda Blvd. (Manhattan Beach); Valley Dr. and Herondo St. (Hermosa Beach)

Mileage
3.5

Type
Rail-Trail

Roughness Rating
2

Surface
Dirt, Wood Chips

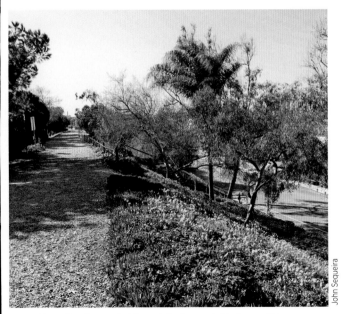

John Sequeira

The soft-surface, pedestrian-only trail connects the towns of Hermosa Beach and Manhattan Beach.

Wood chips give the trail a soft surface through the 24-acre greenbelt sandwiched between Valley Drive and Ardmore Avenue, although Hermosa Beach is installing a firmer surface on a 0.3-mile segment between the Pier Avenue and Eighth Street intersections to make wheelchair use easier.

Eucalyptus and other trees create shady spots along the trail, with other sections grown over with ice plants. Homeowners seeking to beautify their piece of trail provide flowering shrubs and other landscaping. Benches and drinking fountains are located every quarter mile or so.

The northern end of Veterans Parkway heads southwest from a large parking lot just south of Rosecrans Avenue on an access road for the Manhattan Village Shopping and Dining Complex. After passing residential neighborhoods for about a mile, you'll come to busy playing fields at Dorsey Field and Live Oak Park. Another quarter mile takes you to the intersection with Manhattan Beach Boulevard, where you can leave the trail and head west to the beach, accessible in four blocks.

Crossing the intersection, you'll find benches set among seven butterfly totems celebrating the monarchs that are drawn to the local eucalyptus. A wheelchair-accessible parcourse sits between 10th and 11th Streets.

The trail enters Hermosa Beach just past Boundary Place and continues on a 1.7-mile segment through quiet neighborhoods and several parks—including Valley Park and South Park—where you'll find playing fields and gardens with native flora and butterfly habitat.

The trail ends at Herondo Street on the border with Redondo Beach. Heading west for 400 feet on Herondo Street takes you to the The Strand, also known as the Marvin Braude Bike Trail, which rolls for 21 miles along the coast from Pacific Palisades to Torrance.

CONTACT rtc.li/veterans-parkway

PARKING

Parking areas are listed from north to south. *Indicates that at least one accessible parking space is available.*

MANHATTAN BEACH* Manhattan Village entrance access road, 450 feet south of Rosecrans Ave. (33.9004, -118.3956).

MANHATTAN BEACH* 1822–1976 Valley Dr., between 20th Pl. and 17th St., (33.8904, -118.4100).

MANHATTAN BEACH* Valley Dr., between 15th St. and 12th St. (33.8864, -118.4080).

MANHATTAN BEACH* Valley Dr. and 10th Pl. (33.8849, -118.4070).

HERMOSA BEACH* Valley Dr., between 11th St. and Eighth St. (33.8608, -118.3943).

HERMOSA BEACH* South Park, 279 Valley Dr. (33.8575, -118.3947).

Modesto's 2.7-mile Virginia Corridor Trailway is a suburban rail-trail well-used by walkers, runners, bicyclists, and families. Extending between Campus Way to the southwest and Woodrow Avenue to the north, the popular landscaped trail connects to many of the city's residential neighborhoods, schools, parks, churches, and retail and dining establishments.

The trail is built on the former Tidewater Southern Railway corridor, which has been transformed into a premier linear park, trail, and recreational gathering place. The railway provided passenger service through the 1930s, when it transitioned primarily to freight.

The only trailhead and designated parking area is located in a shopping plaza near the midpoint of the trail,

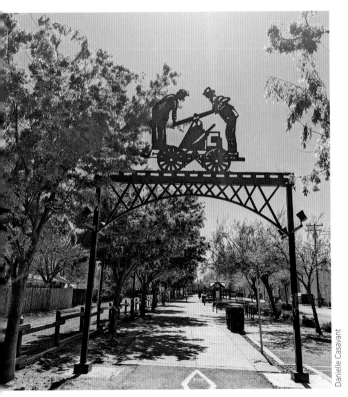

Danielle Casavant

This Modesto trail offers nods to its past as a Tidewater Southern Railway corridor.

County
Stanislaus

Endpoints
Woodrow Ave. and Fremont St. (Modesto); Campus Way and Terminal Ave. (Modesto)

Mileage
2.7

Type
Rail-Trail

Roughness Rating
1

Surface
Asphalt

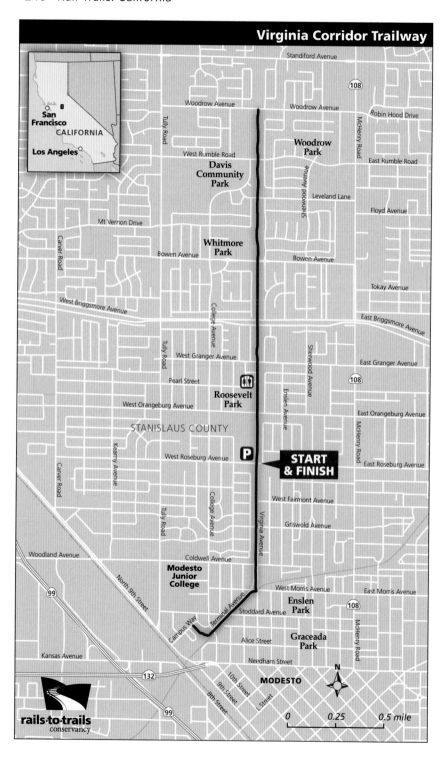

Virginia Corridor Trailway

Standiford Avenue

San Francisco
CALIFORNIA
Los Angeles

Woodrow Avenue

Woodrow Avenue

Robin Hood Drive

Tully Road

McHenry Road

Woodrow
Park

East Rumble Road

West Rumble Road

Davis
Community
Park

Sherwood Avenue

Leveland Lane

Floyd Avenue

Mt Vernon Drive

Whitmore
Park

Carver Road

Bowen Avenue

Bowen Avenue

Tokay Avenue

West Briggsmore Avenue

East Briggsmore Avenue

College Avenue

Tully Road

West Granger Avenue

East Granger Avenue

Sherwood Avenue

Pearl Street

Roosevelt
Park

West Orangeburg Avenue

Enslen Avenue

East Orangeburg Avenue

STANISLAUS COUNTY

McHenry Road

West Roseburg Avenue

P

START
& FINISH

East Roseburg Avenue

Kearny Avenue

Carver Road

Tully Road

West Fairmont Avenue

College Avenue

Griswold Avenue

Virginia Avenue

Woodland Avenue

Coldwell Avenue

Modesto
Junior
College

North 9th Street

99

West Morris Avenue

East Morris Avenue

Terminal Avenue

Enslen
Park

108

Campus Way

Stoddard Avenue

Alice Street

Graceada
Park

McHenry Road

Kansas Avenue

Needham Street

132

8th Street

9th Street

10th Street

L Street

MODESTO

N

99

0   0.25   0.5 mile

rails·to·trails
conservancy

at West Roseburg Avenue. Here, visitors will find signage about the history of the railroad and the region's agricultural roots. Trail users can choose to head north or south for an out-and-back trip. There are many road crossings along the route, but all are well-marked with stop signs and crossing signals.

CONTACT modestogov.com/548/virginia-corridor-trailway

PARKING

One parking location is available roughly midway along the trail. *Indicates that at least one accessible parking space is available.*

MODESTO* 801–921 W. Roseburg Ave. (37.6617, -121.0031).

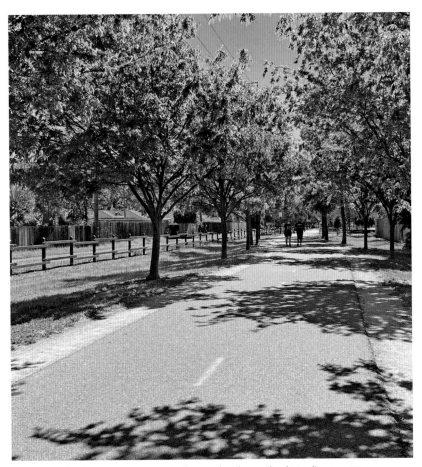

The tree-lined pathway serves as a premier linear park and recreational amenity.   Brandi Horton

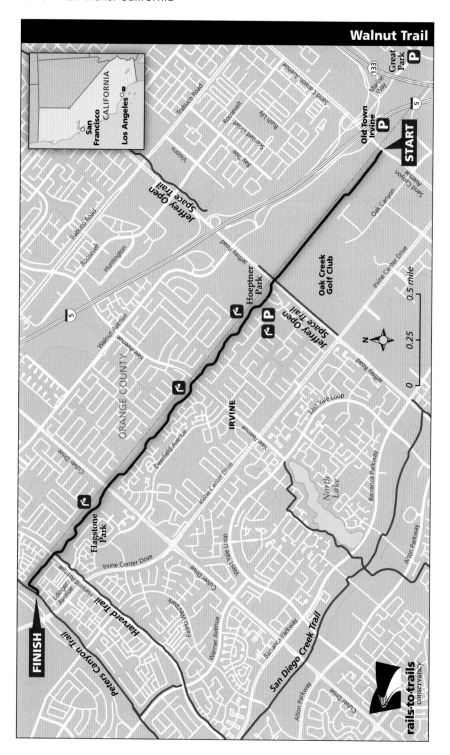

rvine's Walnut Trail shares a wide corridor with an active BNSF Railway line through a section of Orange County that was known for producing oranges and strawberries until the 1970s. While the trail has a distinctly urban feel (the majority is located under power lines), you can still see hints of the area's agricultural past, including several remnant orchards.

The Atchison, Topeka and Santa Fe Railway line originally provided a vital link for transporting iron from the Midwest into the Los Angeles area. In 1971, Amtrak assumed operation of the line, using it to transport passengers between Chicago and Los Angeles. BNSF officially maintains the track and uses it for freight rail, in conjunction with Amtrak and Metrolink passenger service.

The Walnut Trail is a popular commuter trail into central Irvine, one of Southern California's most bike-friendly cities, with many access points along the way. It is also one of the oldest of the city's many trails. Just a 0.3-mile walk

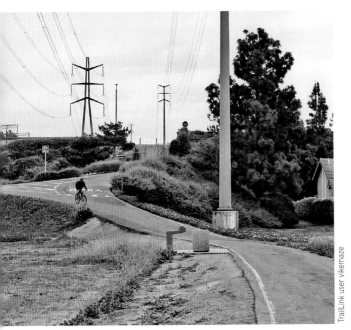

TrailLink user vikemaze

While the trail runs largely beneath power lines, it still offers hints of the area's agricultural past.

County
Orange

Endpoints
Sand Canyon Ave., between Progress and Oak Canyon (Irvine); Peters Canyon Trail, 0.3 mile northwest of Harvard Ave. (Irvine)

Mileage
3.4

Type
Rail-with-Trail

Roughness Rating
1

Surface
Asphalt

from the trail's eastern endpoint is Old Town Irvine—a registered California Historic Landmark—where you can learn about the town's agricultural roots. The public Great Park, east of Old Town Irvine, was built on the former Marine Corps Air Station El Toro and now encompasses sports fields, an Olympic regulation ice rink, and the iconic Great Park Balloon, the first tethered helium balloon in the country.

The trail begins off Sand Canyon Avenue just south of the railroad underpass. This well-maintained, smoothly paved trail follows the tracks northwest. You will cut through a section of the lush Oak Creek Golf Club before reaching Jeffrey Road, beyond which the trail comes to grassy Hoeptner Park, which is a nice spot to rest, stop by the water fountain, or have a picnic (street parking is also available here). From here, the trail crosses some pleasant neighborhoods.

The trail passes underneath Yale Avenue and continues to busy Culver Drive, where another trail overpass carries you across the road. There are access points to the street and sidewalks if you need to connect to sections of town. The trail continues through Flagstone Park toward the end of the trail, providing a rest spot before you make the final push.

A final street crossing at Harvard Avenue offers a connection to the Harvard Trail; another 0.3 mile takes you to the end of the trail, where it intersects with the Peters Canyon Trail.

CONTACT cityofirvine.org/transportation/biking

PARKING

Parking areas are located within Irvine and are listed from east to west. Additionally, limited on-street parking may be found in the neighborhoods surrounding the Harvard Avenue crossing. *Indicates that at least one accessible parking space is available.*

GREAT PARK* Parking Lot 1, 400 feet east of Ridge Valley and Phantom, 0.2 mile southeast of the trail's eastern endpoint (33.6740, -117.7482).

HOEPTNER PARK* Dead end of Hoeptner St., 250 feet east of Touraine Way (33.6860, -117.7763).

TUSTIN METROLINK STATION* Edinger Ave. at Jamboree Plaza, 0.3 mile northwest of the trail's western endpoint (33.7077, -117.8065).

The West County Regional Trail is built along the corridor of the old Petaluma and Santa Rosa Railway, which once carried passengers between Santa Rosa, Petaluma, and Sebastopol. Seamlessly linked with the Joe Rodota Trail (see page 103) in Sebastopol, the rail-trail is part of a developing 2,600-miles-plus Bay Area regional trail network being spearheaded by the Bay Area Trails Collaborative (**railsto trails.org/bay-area**) and Rails-to-Trails Conservancy as a TrailNation™ project to increase safe walking, biking, and trail access for millions of Bay Area residents.

Sweeping rural vistas abound along the trail. Beginning at a junction with the Joe Rodota Trail along CA 116/Gravenstein Highway North, the West County Regional Trail continues north along the highway past lush vineyards and farmland. (Take the Joe Rodota Trail southeast if you want to reach downtown Sebastopol or Santa Rosa instead.)

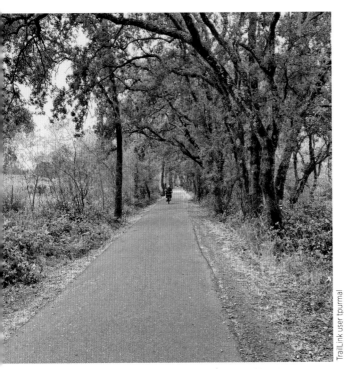

Portions of the pathway traverse oak woodlands and offer prime spots for birding.

TrailLink user tpurmal

County
Sonoma

Endpoints
Joe Rodota Trail at Mill Station Road and CA 116/Gravenstein Hwy. N. (Sebastopol); CA 116/Front St. between Mirabel Road and Second St. (Forestville)

Mileage
5.5

Type
Rail-Trail

Roughness Rating
1–2

Surface
Asphalt, Boardwalk, Gravel

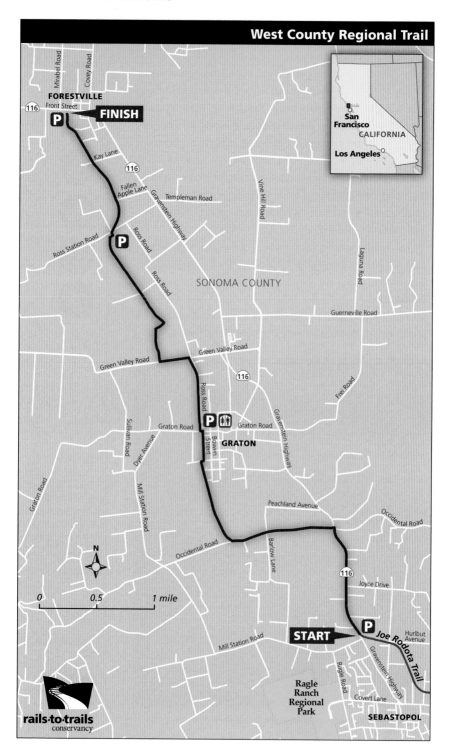

West County Regional Trail

After 1 mile, turn left onto Occidental Road, and go just under another mile until you see the resumption of the off-road trail on your right. Turn onto the trail and continue north 0.7 mile. Turn right onto Grey Street in Graton, then take an immediate left onto Bowen Street. Head 0.2 mile on Bowen Street (note that there are no bike lanes for this stretch). Turn left onto Graton Road, then take an immediate right at the trail directional sign. Continue north on the trail 0.6 mile. Turn left onto Green Valley Road and use the shoulder for about a quarter mile before turning right at the trail directional sign. The paved trail will lead you to an elevated wooden boardwalk. The section from Green Valley Road north for about a half mile is compacted gravel and passes a wastewater treatment plant, but the rest of this last section of the trail passes through beautiful vineyards, picturesque farmland, and orchards.

Roughly 2.2 miles from the resumption of the paved trail at Green Valley Road is a sign for Pajaro Lane in Forestville. Remain on the trail, which crosses another elevated wooden boardwalk and brings you to the small town of Forestville, where you can find picnic tables, an unpaved parking lot, and Forestville's commercial core on CA 116/Front Street.

Note that while horseback riding is permitted for the entirety of the trail, there is no equestrian parking available in the designated trail parking lots.

CONTACT parks.sonomacounty.ca.gov/visit/find-a-park/west-county-regional-trail

PARKING

Parking areas are listed from south to north. *Indicates that at least one accessible parking space is available.*

SEBASTOPOL* Sebastopol Charter School, 1111 Gravenstein Hwy. N. (38.4132, -122.8419); 5 spaces reserved for trail users.

GRATON* Trailhead at Ross and Graton Roads (38.4363, -122.8701); enter parking lot from Graton Road, and exit at Irving St.

ROSS* Ross Station Road Trailhead, 250 feet southwest of Ross Station and Ross Branch Roads (38.4586, -122.8859).

FORESTVILLE CA 116/Front St. Trailhead, gravel lot between Second St. and Mirabel Road (38.4735, -122.8934).

Westside Rails to Trails (Hull Creek to Clavey River)

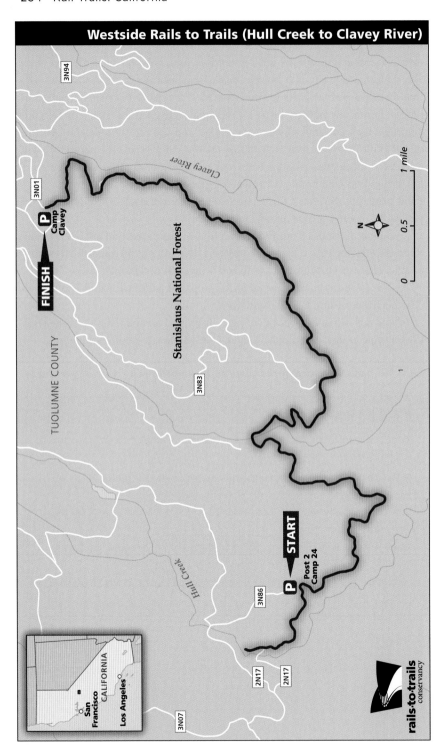

3N94

3N01

Clavey River

P

Camp
Clavey

FINISH

N

1 mile

0.5

0

Stanislaus National Forest

TUOLUMNE COUNTY

3N83

1

P

START

Post 2
Camp 24

3N86

Hull Creek

2N17

2N17

3N07

CALIFORNIA

San
Francisco

Los Angeles

rails-to-trails
conservancy

If you're looking for solitude amid the beautiful, rugged scenery of the Sierra Nevada Mountains, this trail is for you. The Hull Creek segment of the Stanislaus National Forest's Westside Rails to Trails route is off the beaten path, and it's quite possible you'll have the entire trail to yourself. Located in the heart of Stanislaus National Forest, the trail features numbered posts marking points of interest along the old West Side Lumber Company's Hetch Hetchy & Yosemite Valley Railway. (At the Mi-Wok Ranger District office in Mi-Wok Village, you can pick up a brochure corresponding to the trail's numbered posts, as well as maps of the trail and the general area.)

The trail is passable by mountain bike, but be prepared for a rough ride, including carrying your bike through washouts and over fallen trees. The trail is great for hiking, but it's 9 miles one-way, so make sure you come prepared for the round-trip or arrange for a pickup. Bring a compass and a map, as finding the trailhead isn't easy; in places, the railroad corridor itself is not obvious, even

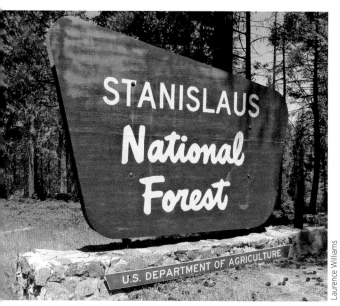

The Westside Rails to Trails route is tucked into the heart of Stanislaus National Forest.

Laurence Williams

County
Tuolumne

Endpoints
FR 3N86 (Long Barn);
FR 3N01 (Long Barn)

Mileage
9

Type
Rail-Trail

Roughness Rating
3

Surface
Ballast, Dirt

when you're on it. Equestrian use is permitted on the entirety of the trail. You can drive a motocross vehicle/ATV (50 inches wide or less) on the road/trail until you reach Post 5, although there is no parking there.

The western endpoint officially begins 0.4 mile south of the crossing of Hull Creek and Forest Route 2N17, but it's best to drive another mile south on FR 3N86 and park at Post 2, the site of an old logging camp (Camp 24) that was once a busy hub for the railroad. Here, several Forest Service roads—which may not appear on a road map—intersect. Once you park, head south on the trail, which follows FR 3N86.

At about 2.5 miles, you will reach Posts 4 and 5. Just beyond this point, the trail emerges into a meadow called Boney Flat. Post 11 marks the beginning of the Trout Creek Spur. The last mile of the trail has a moderately steep climb, then evens out as it approaches an intersection with FR 3N01 at Camp Clavey, an old railroad logging camp and remote U.S. Forest Service fire station. While little remains of the camp, several dispersed campsites with day-use parking are available.

For more adventure, head toward the Clavey River on a side trail from Post 11, near Buffalo Landing. The river makes for a great place to cool off during warm summer afternoons, but the real attraction is the old 75-foot Clavey River trestle. The trestle burned down long ago, but its foundation still remains, a testament to the rich railroad history of the Sierra Nevada.

CONTACT rtc.li/stanislaus-nf

PARKING

Parking areas are located within Long Barn and are listed from west to east. * *Indicates that at least one accessible parking space is available.*

WEST FR 3N86, at the intersection of FR 2N03 and FR 2N31Y, near Post 2/Camp 24 (38.0374, -120.0893); horse trailer parking available. The intersection of FR 2N03 and FR 2N31Y may not show up on a road map; instead, follow the GPS coordinates and look for the (second, southern) intersection of FR 3N86 and FR 2N17. Start from Post 2 and head southeast on the trail.

EAST Camp Clavey Road 3N56Y, off FR 3N01, just north of the Clavey River, 5 miles south of Hull Creek Campground and 15 miles southeast of Long Barn (38.0719, -120.0260); horse trailer parking available.

Tucked away in sparsely populated Tuolumne County, this portion of the Stanislaus National Forest's Westside Rails to Trails route is a hidden treasure, combining spectacular scenery and a representation of an amazing feat of railway construction.

The county's timber industry was in full gear at the turn of the 20th century. An impressive sawmill was built at that time, and the West Side Lumber Company constructed its own narrow-gauge railroad—the Hetch Hetchy & Yosemite Valley Railway—to bring timber to the mill. The initial stretch of the mainline grade, constructed without the benefit of bulldozers and loaders, was blasted into an extremely steep and rocky canyon. As you walk along the rail-trail, you cannot fail to be impressed by what the workers accomplished. Interpretive panels along the trail provide information about the area's logging history and Indigenous heritage.

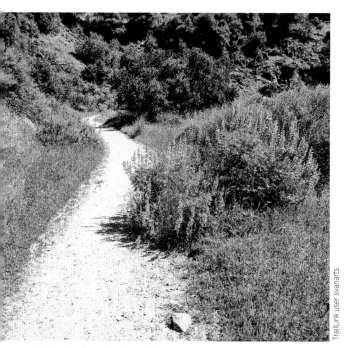

TrailLink user svanarts

Lupine bushes and other wildflowers adorn this passage through Stanislaus National Forest.

County
Tuolumne

Endpoints
Buchanan Road and Mira Monte Road (Tuolumne); FR 1N04 and Fish Hatchery Road (Twain Harte)

Mileage
5.5

Type
Rail-Trail

Roughness Rating
3

Surface
Crushed Stone, Dirt

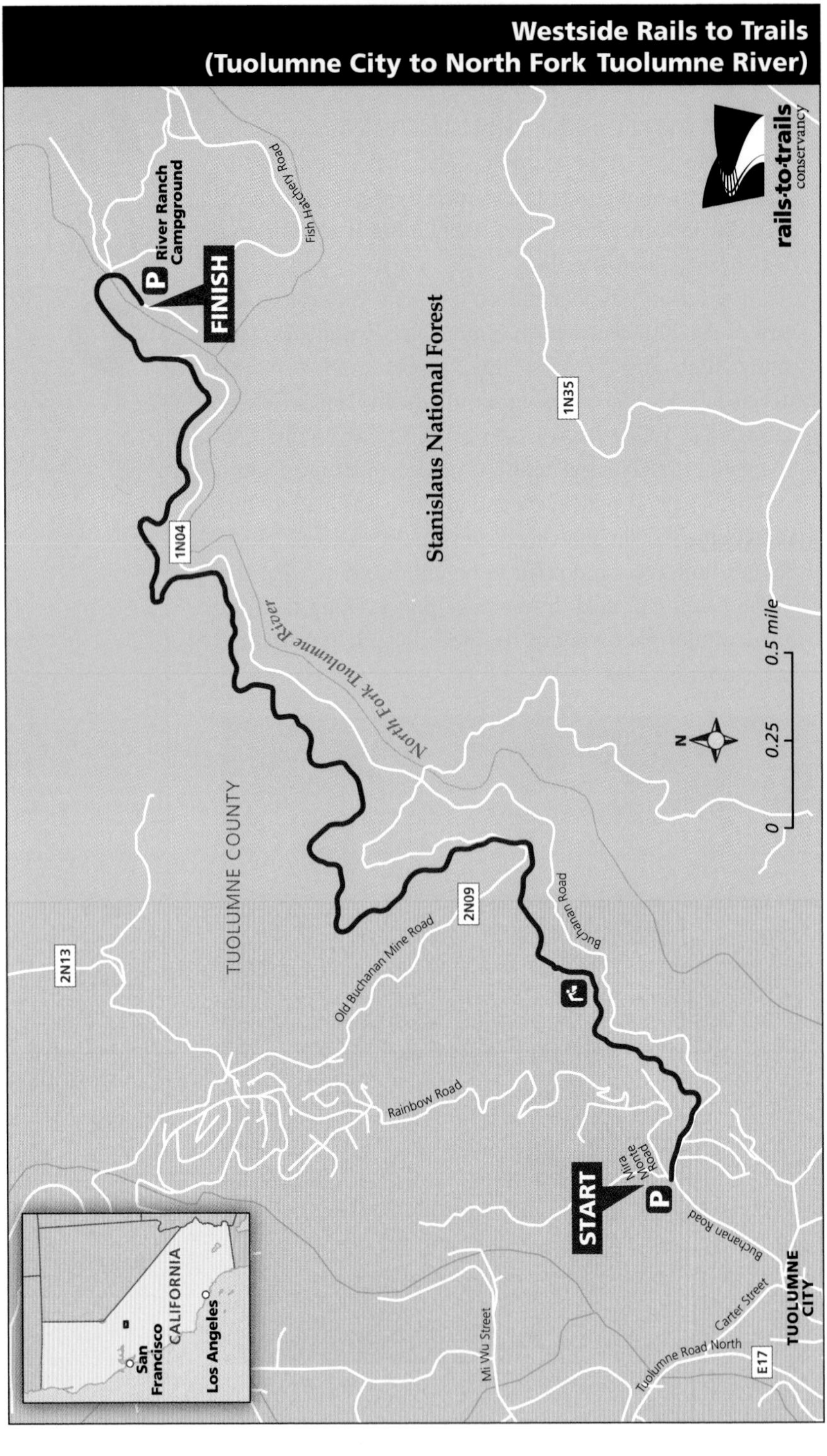

Westside Rails to Trails
(Tuolumne City to North Fork Tuolumne River)

rails·to·trails
conservancy

River Ranch Campground

FINISH

Fish Hatchery Road

Stanislaus National Forest

1N35

1N04

North Fork Tuolumne River

0   0.25   0.5 mile

N

TUOLUMNE COUNTY

2N09

Old Buchanan Mine Road

Buchanan Road

2N13

Rainbow Road

START

Mira Monte Road

Buchanan Road

Carter Street

Mi Wu Street

Tuolumne Road North

E17

TUOLUMNE CITY

CALIFORNIA

San Francisco

Los Angeles

Located next to a small parking lot and a residential street, the unsigned Tuolumne City trailhead at the western terminus is unassuming. (Note that equestrian parking is available here; equestrian use is permitted for the entirety of the trail.) At first, the trail is surrounded by trees on both sides, but after less than a half mile, it opens up to spectacular views. On your right, you see a gaping canyon, with layers of rolling, tree-covered hills beyond. After another half mile, you come to a picnic bench and, shortly after, the only water fountain on the trail. (It is a good idea to bring water and protection from the sun.) At the 1-mile mark, you see the old rails and ties that run from this point through the end of the trail, adding to its beauty and character. The dramatic scenery continues as the path traverses the steep canyon. Patches of wildflowers that grow between the narrow-gauge tracks appear in the springtime, making this rail-trail all the more beautiful.

At certain points, the path becomes slightly narrow and rocky. About 5 miles in, you'll come upon a thick patch of trees that seems impassable, at which point you won't be able to continue walking parallel with the rails. From here, you can return the way you came or veer right and descend the steep switchbacks for about a half mile to a main road (Fish Hatchery Road/Buchanan Road/Forest Route 1N04). Turn left here and walk along the road on a half-mile looping route that will bring you to the entrance of the River Ranch Campground.

It is possible to leave a car at the campground before setting out, then shuttle to the trailhead (note that there is a day-use fee at the campground). If you are on a mountain bike and want a speedier return to the Tuolumne City trailhead parking lot, you can cycle westward about 4.25 miles on Fish Hatchery Road/Buchanan Road/FR 1N04. This route is a steep climb, and while the two-lane road is lightly trafficked, there is no biking lane and it's narrow at some points, so use caution.

CONTACT rtc.li/stanislaus-nf

PARKING

Parking areas are listed from west to east. *Indicates that at least one accessible parking space is available.*

TUOLUMNE Tuolumne City trailhead, Buchanan Road/FR 1N04 and Mira Monte Road (37.9731, -120.2271).

TWAIN HARTE River Ranch Campground, 20900 Fish Hatchery Road, 0.1 mile southwest of FR 1N04 (37.9941, -120.1813).

Index

Rails-to-Trails Conservancy (RTC) is a nonprofit organization working to build a nation connected by trails. We reimagine public spaces to create safe ways for everyone to walk, bike, and be active outdoors. Since 1986, RTC has worked from coast to coast, helping to transform unused rail corridors and other rights-of-way into vibrant public places, ensuring a better future for America made possible by trails and the connections they inspire.

We know trails improve lives, engage communities, create opportunities, and inspire movement. And we know these opportunities are possible only with the help of our passionate members and supporters across the country. Learn how you can support RTC and discover the benefits of membership at **railstotrails.org/support.**

Rails-to-Trails Conservancy is a 501(c)(3) nonprofit organization, and contributions are tax-deductible.

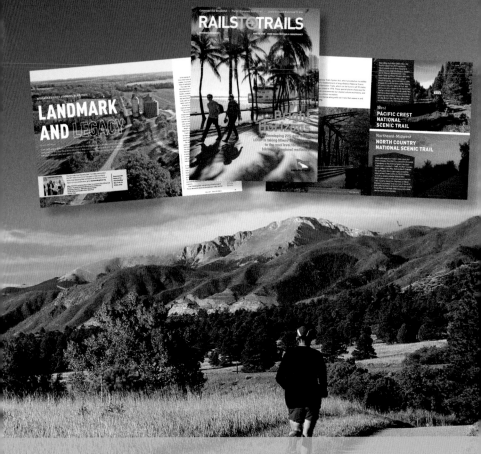

rails·to·trails
conservancy

SHARE THE TRAIL

Be nice.
Trails are for everyone.

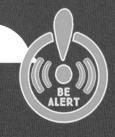

BE ALERT

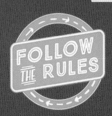

USE SAFE SPEEDS

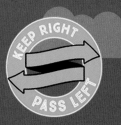

KEEP RIGHT
PASS LEFT

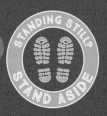

STANDING STILL?
STAND ASIDE

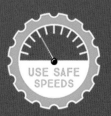

FOLLOW THE RULES

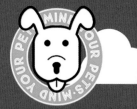

MIND YOUR PET

Calling all trail users! Rails-to-Trails Conservancy
challenges YOU to be the best you can be on America's pathways!
Remember—safe + fun = a great time for everyone!

#sharethetrail

Visit **railstotrails.org/sharethetrail** for more.

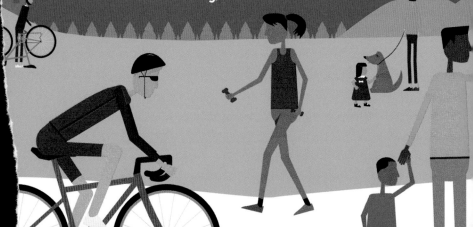

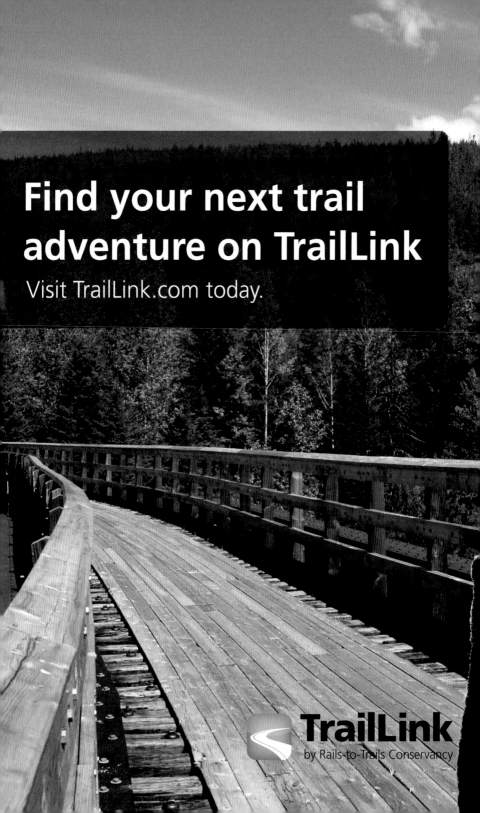